Homemade Smoothies
for
Mother and Baby

Homemade Smoothies

for

Mother and Baby

Over 200 Healthy
Fruit and Green Smoothies
for Pregnancy, Nursing and
Baby's First Years

Kristine Miles

Published in the U.S. by:
Ulysses Press
P.O. Box 3440
Berkeley, CA 94703
www.ulyssespress.com

ISBN13: 978-1-61243-477-3
Library of Congress Control Number: 2015937558

10 9 8 7 6 5 4 3 2 1

Acquisitions Editor: Katherine Furman
Project Editor: Alice Riegert
Managing Editor: Claire Chun
Editor: Laurie Dunne
Proofreader: Lauren Harrison
Index: Sayre Van Young
Front cover design: TG Design
Interior design: Jake Flaherty
Cover artwork: all images from shuterstock.com; glass © Madlen; sippy cup ©
    Alexey Arkhipov; strawberry © Denis Tabler; blueberry; Dlonlsvera; kiwi ©
    ranglzzz; broccoli © photosync; cucumber © plyaraya

NOTE TO READERS: This book has been written and published strictly for
informational and educational purposes only. It is not intended to serve as
medical advice or to be any form of medical treatment. You should always
consult with your physician before altering or changing any aspect of your
medical treatment. Do not stop or change any prescription medications
without the guidance and advice of your physician. Any use of the information
in this book is made on the reader's good judgment and is the reader's sole
responsibility. This book is not intended to diagnose or treat any medical
condition and is not a substitute for a physician. This book is independently
authored and published and no sponsorship or endorsement of this book by,
and no affiliation with, any trademarked brands or other products mentioned
within is claimed or suggested. All trademarks that appear in ingredient lists
and elsewhere in this book belong to their respective owners and are used here
for informational purposes only. The authors and publishers encourage readers
to patronize the quality brands mentioned and pictured in this book.

This book is dedicated to my mum, my biggest supporter. I know you are clapping and cheering for me in spirit. I hope you are at peace and know you are loved and dearly missed every single day.

Contents

Introduction

In July 2013, my husband and I were blessed with the arrival of our daughter, Emily. Her journey into our lives was not without its dramas. First, with unexplained infertility, it took over 3 years to conceive, followed by finding out she had a birth defect of her abdomen at 12 weeks with risks of associated serious medical problems, *and* being advised she would require around 6 months in the NICU (neonatal intensive care unit) at a hospital 2 hours from our home.

Knowing what was ahead of us, I worked hard at having a very healthy pregnancy and breastfeeding period, to ensure Emily had the best start in life possible. Contrary to the doom and gloom presented while I was pregnant, she was born strong and healthy, and spent just 8 weeks in the hospital, defying the odds and amazing the doctors looking after her, with no infections, no breathing assistance, no formula feeds, and no fortified feeds—her medicine was lots of love and my breast milk.

Emily's conception was all thanks to the wonderful guidance of my natural fertility specialist naturopath, using herbal medicine and tweaking my already healthy way of eating. My excellent health, and that of Emily, had a lot to do with how much effort I put into my diet, and smoothies played a big role in this picture. I have been drinking green smoothies since 2007, and my passion for the humble green drink resulted in the publication of my first book *The Green Smoothie Bible,* published in 2012, and *Green Smoothies for Every Season,* published in 2013.

This publication is a smoothie handbook for all things maternal, from preconception to pregnancy to breastfeeding and introducing solids to your children. The smoothies are inspired by the nutritional requirements recommended for each stage, what tastes great, the latest research and guidelines, and my personal journey, plus the journeys of the wonderful, smoothie-drinking mamas I surveyed. I hope you enjoy *Homemade Smoothies for Mother and Baby* as much as I enjoyed writing it.

So Why Smoothies?

Smoothies, to me, are the ultimate fast food but even better—a healthy fast food (bypassing ice-cream-laden smoothies!). Smoothies are quick to prepare, the cleanup is as simple as rinsing the blender jug and leaving it upside down to air dry, and they are easy to transport. I am a fan of a smoothie for breakfast and often take mine to work with me in a glass jar with a lid (tomato sauce jars or mason jars are perfect). I find that a half-liter/1-pint smoothie sustains me through to lunchtime, so it's perfect for me. My husband gets hungry again sooner, but that's the difference with our bodies, as not everyone is the same when it comes to digestion, metabolism, and blood sugar maintenance.

Smoothies can be made purely for pleasure, filling enough to be a meal, designed to optimize nutrient availability, structured to serve a particular purpose, or all of these. In my book *The Green Smoothie Bible*, I created hundreds of green smoothie recipes that

I categorized for cardiovascular health, blood sugar regulation, weight loss, hormone health, mood, bowel health, and more.

Additionally, smoothies can be light like juice, made with rich ingredients for fun and decadent, dessert-like drinks, or as simple two- or three-ingredient smoothies.

Green Smoothies

Though I am well known for creating and writing about green smoothies, the smoothies in this book are not all green ones: Some of them are and some have an option to be. Green smoothies, for those who don't know, are smoothies with leafy greens blended into them. Traditionally, they are vegan smoothies with raw leafy greens, sweet raw fruit, and water for the "purist"; however, there is no rule that says you can't use milk or add fats, vegetables, or cooked fruits. Green smoothies will not appeal to everyone, but I would love to convince you to give them a try! The very point of green smoothies is to get more greens into your diet.

Mix Up Your Greens

If using greens in smoothies regularly, make sure that you don't use the same green all the time. Greens contain substances called "secondary plant metabolites" that in small amounts are harmless, but in large amounts can be harmful or unpleasant, such as the oxalic acid in Swiss chard and spinach or essential oils in herbs, and other greens have tannins, nitrates, phytates, or saponins. I can tell if I have been eating too much of the same green, because I cease desiring green smoothies and I feel a bit queasy mid-morning after having one at breakfast. In the wild, these substances in plants are a defense mechanism to prevent devastation by predators. Hence, animals naturally rotate their food sources and so should we.

BUT WHY MORE GREENS?

- Greens are alkaline, rich in antioxidant pigments like chlorophyll that are very cleansing, and are very low calorie.

- Greens are rich in vitamins, particularly beta-carotene (the precursor to vitamin A) and vitamin C, and minerals such as calcium, magnesium, and iron.

- Greens contain amino acids that are the building blocks of protein. Spinach has 30 percent of its calories as protein compared to milk at 23 percent and beef at 50 percent. Cooking destroys protein by 50 percent, so 100g of cooked beef is similar to around 80g of raw spinach for available protein content.

- Greens contain fiber and hence are great for the health of our bowel—a happy bowel is a happy body! Fiber blended into tiny pieces actually makes it do a better job in your gut.

- Blending greens makes it easier to eat a larger volume of greenery than by chewing, makes greenery easier to digest, and ruptures cell membranes, releasing nutrients that may otherwise not be released by chewing.

- The addition of greens to a smoothie satiates the appetite due to the additional fiber and the extra nutrients. Fiber is filling, and nutrient-poor, low-fiber food frequently leads to overconsumption that may lead to obesity.

- Any smoothie can have a handful of greens thrown in, with the greens or other ingredients influencing the color of the smoothie. Don't let the green color of a green smoothie put you off, because the pairing of greens and sweet fruit is perfect and the taste delicious! However, a smoothie with chocolate or berries will hide the green color well, which is handy if you have an adult or child funny about drinking something green! The main thing with green smoothies is to make them sweet enough to balance the bitterness of blended greens.

So Why Smoothies and Not Juices?

Juices, like smoothies, can be nourishing drinks rich in vitamins, minerals, and antioxidants, particularly if they are homemade. They are, however, void of fiber, so unless you are drinking huge quantities often, they are not filling. Moreover, the lack of fiber means the natural sugars from the fruits or sweet vegetables used are quickly absorbed into the bloodstream, potentially spiking blood sugar. Fiber slows this process for a sustained release of energy, which is better for blood sugar regulation and is more successful at satisfying hunger.

Juices and smoothies can have similar calorie content; however, juices are often drunk with a meal or close to a meal, so they are usually an unnecessary addition of carbohydrate-based calories to the diet, and not a good option if trying to lose weight. (Unless the juice is a non-sweet veggie juice, then the calorie factor is negligible but it still won't be filling). Conversely, smoothies are filling, fiber rich, and frequently consumed as a food, rather than accompanying food. I think of smoothies as a food, not a drink—you just happen to drink them!

CHAPTER 1

The Art and Science of Smoothies

Making smoothies is really very easy, when all that is required is to put ingredients in a blender and flick on a switch. However, making smoothies taste great and serving their purpose can be more challenging!

Flavor

If your smoothies are not delicious, you won't drink them frequently. Smoothies may be a drink, but they are really a blended food. To make smoothies taste great, you need to balance flavor and texture, including sweet, salty, sour, spicy, and bitter, but not in equal proportions. There will be dominant flavors that need balancing by the others—just like Napolitano and Bolognese pasta sauces will be very bland without salt, smoothies come to life by adding a teaspoon of sugar for sweetness, a pinch of chili or cracked pepper for spice, a dash of curry powder for bitterness, and a splash of vinegar for acidity.

Smoothies will have a dominant sweet flavor, but they can run into trouble being too sweet, or too bitter if making green smoothies or smoothies with cacao. Bitterness can be remedied with a little salt, sweetness, or warmth. This is why green smoothies are best made with sweet fruit, and a pinch of salt in a cacao smoothie is magic for enhancing flavor. If your smoothie is too sweet due to the fruit or too much extra sweetener, try adding some acid from lemon or lime juice, as sweet and sour are classically paired. Conversely, if your smoothie is too sour, add something sweet. Fruit will generally provide some sweetness and sourness to varying degrees, with very ripe bananas and lemons being at either end of the spectrum. Spice in smoothies can come from the use of ingredients like ginger, cinnamon, or cardamom. Too much hot spice can also be settled with extra sweetener.

I recommend sweet fruit be used in smoothies so that the primary sweetener comes from fruit and not added sweeteners. There is a lot of anti-sugar business going on these days and while I generally agree that is a good thing, I do feel it goes too far with fruit seen as something evil that shouldn't be consumed. Fruit is not like pure sugar. It contains sugar (glucose and fructose), sure, but it also contains vitamins, minerals, antioxidants, and most importantly fiber! Fiber, particularly soluble fiber, helps to slow the digestion of the sugars in fruit, so blood sugars don't spike, sending you up and then quickly down looking for your next fix—which is what concentrated sweets do like sodas and chocolates. So please enjoy eating fruit, and if you do wish to limit it to one or two pieces a day, then in your smoothie is perfect.

Temperature and Consistency

Smoothies also require the right temperature and texture; however, this is often unique to an individual. Some prefer thick, icy-cold smoothies, others like thinner, room temperature smoothies. There isn't much doubt, however, that smoothies should be smooth—it's all in the name after all! A smoothie with lumps and bits through it isn't very pleasant, and hence why it's a good idea to invest in a good-quality, high-speed blender if smoothies are to be a regular fixture in your diet, as they make a lovely, silky smoothie and as an appliance they have longevity. Examples of good blenders are the brands Blendtec and Vitamix, which are readily available in shops and online. My choice is Thermomix, which is a multi-function appliance that works as a high-speed blender, food processer, and also cooks. It is German and is available via direct sales in most Western countries except the United States. Less expensive blenders still work but results aren't as good in terms of mouthfeel, and they can struggle with ice cubes, frozen fruit, dates, whole nuts, pineapple cores, etc. They will also break down quickly with regular, particularly daily, use.

If you prefer a thicker smoothie, there are several things to keep in mind. Some ingredients act as thickening agents, such as chia seeds, oats, or fruits high in pectin like apples, blueberries, and plums. Also, adding extra fiber and fat from items like coconut flesh, whole nuts and seeds, or oils will help bulk up a smoothie, and obviously, using less liquid will as well. Smoothies using frozen ingredients will have the illusion of being thicker and creamier due to air held in the crushed icicles—until they melt!

The Process

The process of putting all the ingredients in the blender to me is quite simple and I don't believe a particular order is necessary. If your blender is powerful enough and it has smooth sides (like the Thermomix jug, for instance), everything is combined quickly with no assistance needed. Many blender jugs have ridges on the inside, and the use of a "tamper" is needed. A tamper is a plastic probe that you stick through the hole in the lid to push ingredients down to assist the mixing process. Less expensive blenders don't have as much power or tampers, so ingredients should be sliced smaller, and sometimes a larger-sized smoothie needs to be done in stages, such as blending dates with the liquid, then adding fruit. The following will be assumed for all recipes:

- Fruits like banana, pineapple, melons, and papaya are to be peeled.

- Removal of apple and pear cores is optional and not necessary in high-speed blenders, but do remove the stem.

- All fruits should be ripe: bananas with brown spots, soft stone fruit, etc.

- Fruit like peaches, apricots, and mangoes should have the stone removed.

- Fruits like cherries, cantaloupes, honeydew melons, and papayas should have seeds removed.

- Citrus should have most of its seeds removed, as otherwise the smoothie will be quite bitter (albeit very medicinal!).

- Soft fruit should be portioned so that pieces are about a quarter- to half-cup in size, such as halved bananas, halved stone fruits, cut melon and pineapple, etc.

- Very soft fruits like mango and avocado don't require worrying about size.

- Harder items like celery, beet, and apple should be at least half the size of soft fruits.

- With the use of greens, such as Swiss chard, kale, or parsley, they should be as fresh as possible, well cleaned, and tough stalks removed.

- The leafy green suggested for green smoothies can be substituted to suit your availability of greens, and the suggested amount can be decreased or increased according to your preference—the more experienced green smoothie drinker will handle a greater proportion of greenery.

- With added sweeteners, the one suggested is for taste purposes. Feel free to substitute for another, should you prefer, or use none at all.

- If "sweeten to taste" is listed, possible options are medjool dates, agave, honey, coconut nectar, maple syrup, rice malt syrup, or stevia. More about sweeteners later in this chapter.

- Frozen ingredients should be no larger than ice cubes from home freezer trays.

Liquids in Smoothies

Recipes will call for water, coconut water, milk, juice, or cooled tea.

Dairy milk—If not dairy intolerant or not avoiding it for other reasons (see preconception and postnatal chapters), please source full-fat, organic, unhomogenized milk. Organic means the milk won't have pesticide residues in it, will be more nutritious from cows feeding on non-chemically treated pastures, and is a more ethical choice. Homogenization means the milk is mechanically mixed at a high speed, so the cream is dispersed through the milk and doesn't separate—this changes the structure of the milk fat and renders it more difficult to digest. Furthermore, the fat in milk is present to aid the absorption of fat-soluble nutrients like vitamins A, D, E, and K, and the minerals calcium and magnesium.

Non-dairy milk—Non-dairy options of milk may include almond, coconut, oat, rice, and soy. However, I don't recommend soy as it is largely a genetically modified crop and an unhealthy option for preconception, pregnancy, lactation, and children, due to its reproductive-hormone and thyroid-disruptive properties, and its high anti-nutrient content. (Anti-nutrients such as phytates bind with minerals, rendering them poorly absorbed, particularly zinc and iron, which are both very important through all stages presented. Other anti-nutrients are enzyme inhibitors, which interfere with soy's digestion and can lead to upset tummies.) Nuts, seeds, legumes, and grains all contain these "anti-nutrients"; however, soy is the one to avoid due to its numerous adverse properties, and it's a difficult legume to get rid of them in (and hence why traditional cultures like the Japanese ferment soy before use). However, making milks from nuts and seeds like almond and sunflower requires a simple soaking method to reduce anti-nutrient content. Plant-based milks can be bought commercially but they will be pasteurized (heat-treated), which will affect the nutritional profile, and they don't taste as nice as homemade milks.

Homemade Almond Milk

If you would prefer to make your own almond milk for recipes in this book, then the following recipe is perfect and one I have used for many years. You can use commercially prepared almond milk, but it will taste a little different and not be as pure or nutritious. You will need a nut milk bag or straining cloth, such as a muslin.   Yield: 5 cups

1 cup raw almonds

¼ teaspoon salt

filtered water, for soaking

5 cups (1.25 liters) filtered water, for blending

1. Soak the almonds in a glass or ceramic bowl for 24 hours with the salt and enough filtered water to cover the almonds by about an inch or two. Try to change the soak water after 12 hours or so, especially in hot weather.

2. Drain and rinse the soaked almonds well. Place with 5 cups filtered water into your blender bowl with the soaked almonds and blend on high speed for 90 seconds.

3. Place the nut milk bag over a bowl of appropriate size to catch the milk and pour the blended mixture into the top of the bag. Tighten the strings and massage the mixture to help separate the milk from the remaining fiber. Don't squeeze your bag too hard or you may burst the seams and squash fiber through. If using a straining cloth lay it over the bowl, pour the blended almonds on top, gather up the sides, and assist the straining by gently massaging as described above.

4. Store milk in glass jars in your fridge, and use within 3 days. You can make the milk richer by soaking more almonds to the same amount of water, but it can get expensive. Recipe may be halved if 5 cups of almond milk won't be necessary or consumed within 3 days.

Water—Many of us in the Western world take the availability of clean drinking water for granted: It simply comes out of the tap and it's cheap. But it's not just water that comes out of the tap.

Water will carry small amounts of naturally occurring minerals such as calcium, magnesium, sodium, and potassium. For tap water to be "safe" to drink from, it must be treated to get rid of organisms that could poison us. You may be surprised to know that water is commonly treated with chlorine or chloramines, lime, and aluminum sulfate. Some parts of the world add fluoride to water, and tap water can contain traces of heavy metals and drugs such as the contraceptive pill.

Now that I have turned you off tap water, I am not suggesting you buy bottled water instead—this is unnecessarily expensive, is frequently no better than tap water, and it's not ideal to drink water that is stored in plastic either. Instead, I recommend you get the best water filter you can. Filters are rated according to the size of particle they can filter out, the smaller the better, and will be measured in microns. Less than 0.1 micron is what you should aim for, which is microfiltration, but even better is ultrafiltration below 0.01 micron. This may be in the form of an under-sink unit that filters everything that comes out of the tap, or there are various countertop reservoirs with filter systems—some just filter, and some add minerals like calcium and magnesium back into the water. Unless you have a good reverse-osmosis unit, home filters won't remove fluoride, and the filters that do claim to remove fluoride are not very effective, and can leave traces of aluminum in the filtered water.

Coconut water, milk, and cream—Coconut water, milk, and cream are different liquids. Coconut water comes from the center of a fresh coconut (preferably a young Thai coconut, also known as a drinking coconut) and is clear/opaque white in color and sweet. Coconut milk and cream are made from blending coconut flesh with water and separating the fiber (which can be turned into coconut flour). Coconut cream naturally has a higher fat content than coconut milk and will have the richest impact in a smoothie, followed by milk and then water. Coconut water is much sweeter than cream or milk, however, and can be used as a sweetener. Packaged coconut water is an alternative to using drinking coconuts, but please use preservative-free and unsweetened varieties. For more on coconuts, see page 43.

Yogurt—Yogurt is another lovely addition to smoothies. Please source dairy yogurt that is organic and full fat for the same reasons listed for dairy milk. Additionally, it's best to use natural yogurt to avoid unhealthy added sweeteners such as white sugar, high fructose corn syrup, and fruit juice concentrates that are also high in fructose. Many yogurts on the market these days do not resemble pure yogurt, with fat removed and gums added to simulate the texture of the real thing—not to mention artificial sweeteners, and additives such as artificial flavorings and colors. These have no place in our bodies nor those of our children. Better to add some raw honey (not for babies under 1) or pure maple syrup to some natural yogurt than to buy a pre-sweetened variety. Even better and cheaper is to make your own yogurt from organic milk.

As an alternative to dairy, coconut and soy yogurts are available. I don't recommend soy, as already discussed, but coconut can be a lovely substitute, albeit a lot more expensive. Yogurt, though it may look thick in a pot, will blend into a smoothie somewhat like a liquid. It will be a creamier addition to a smoothie than milk and will also add sourness. This can be useful to tone down very sweet fruits like very ripe mangoes and bananas. Conversely, avoid using ingredients with yogurt that are also very tart, such as lemons. Berries are often somewhat sour; however, they partner beautifully with yogurt provided it's balanced with sufficient sweetness.

Milk kefir, which is a fermented milk and like a cross between milk and yogurt, is rich in beneficial bacteria and is given as an alternative option in recipes that include both milk and yogurt.

Juice—Some recipes call for juices to be used as part of the entire liquid base. Citrus juices can simply be squeezed by hand in a citrus juicer. Vegetables such as carrots, beets, fennel, and celery can be juiced in a fast centrifugal or slow masticating juicer. The former is quicker, but the latter makes a more nutritious juice with less waste.

Teas—Another option for smoothie bases are herbal teas, which will add definite flavor and will be used for this purpose and/or its nutritional benefit. Kombucha is a fermented tea that can be homemade or bought commercially. Many who use it regularly tout it as being an excellent tonic for general well-being and for gut health. I have suggested it in one recipe, though regular users are welcome to add it to other recipes if desired. It can be strong tasting with a sour element to it, and may, in my opinion, negatively alter the pleasurable taste that a smoothie should ideally have.

RECIPE TIPS FOR LIQUIDS

If a specific type of milk is suggested in a recipe, it is for flavor and/or its nutritional influence. Feel free to substitute different milk, but bear in mind it may alter the flavor of the smoothie than the one intended, and will also alter the intended nutritional goal—such as the use of almond milk plus peanut butter, which ensures that complete protein (all essential amino acids) is present in the smoothie. If "milk of choice" is listed, please use whatever milk you prefer. However, coconut milk, coconut cream, coconut water, yogurt, or water will be suggested in recipes independently of "milk."

Vegetables in Smoothies

In my recipes, vegetables with excellent nutrient and functional profiles will be frequent inclusions.

Beets—Recipes will indicate raw or cooked beets. Nutritionally, the betalain pigments in beets are destroyed by the cooking process, and given these are liver-friendly substances, smoothies that are aimed at boosting liver function will contain raw beets. Other recipes have the option of raw or cooked. Cooking beets will enhance the sweetness a little and make for easier blending. Steaming is the preferred cooking method, as it will retain nutrients better than boiling. Beets are also lactogenic (breastmilk supportive) vegetables.

Carrots—Carrots are rich in beta-carotene (the precursor to vitamin A) and also lactogenic. My recommendation is to steam for addition to smoothies, though raw is also an option, and carrot juice is listed for some recipes. Organic carrots are highly recommended, not just for avoiding chemicals, but they taste a lot better.

Sweet potato and pumpkin—Also very rich in beta-carotene, these root veggies can be used in pureed form or steamed pieces. If using canned puree, please ensure it is only sweet potato or pumpkin with no additives or sweeteners.

Celery—Celery has a distinctive taste for certain flavor pairings and has diuretic properties, and hence is useful for conditions involving swelling.

Fennel—Also a distinctive-flavored vegetable, fennel (including the bulb, tops, and seeds) are of particular benefit to breastfeeding mothers for maintaining or building milk supply. Some recipes call for ground fennel or fennel tea. Both will use the seeds. One teaspoon makes one cup of tea, and to grind, use a spice grinder or mortar and pestle.

TIME-SAVING TIP

Beets, carrot, pumpkin, and sweet potato also suit freezing after being steamed. They can then be added to smoothies frozen or they thaw out nicely. I highly recommend having a supply of these vegetables in ice-cube-sized pieces, steamed then frozen in ziplock bags. Thaw the amount you need in the fridge the night before and your smoothie is a simple process with ready-to-use ingredients the next day. Storing vegetables like this in the freezer is also a sensible thing to do should you have an excess of any of these vegetables, or if you buy in bulk at a great price but know you will struggle to eat them all while still fresh.

Grains in Smoothies

Three grains are listed in some smoothie recipes. They have nutritional profiles of use to maternal and child health, and they also add bulk to a smoothie as an alternative to fruits or veggies. They also happen to be gluten-free, which is important for preconception, and whether you are gluten intolerant or not, you will be able to enjoy my recipes that include these ingredients.

Oats—Oats may be added to smoothies in raw form or cooked in the form of cooled porridge. Soaking overnight or cooking will aid digestibility and this is how I recommend they be used. It is not uncommon for porridge or Bircher muesli to be well tolerated but not raw muesli, which can upset tummies and cause gas. Some raw oats can leave a bitter taste and an unpleasant mouthfeel when blended raw, but some don't, so it will be up to you to experiment to see what is more palatable for you personally. Porridge makes a nicer, smoother smoothie but is less convenient than throwing in raw oats. The solution to this, if you are likely to use porridge regularly in your smoothies, is to cook up a decent-sized batch and freeze half-cup portions. Then simply thaw in the fridge the night before you intend to use them. Oats are a source of manganese, biotin, vitamin B1, magnesium, chromium, zinc, calcium, and protein. They are also a well-known lactogenic food for breastfeeding mothers.

Note that oats are not strictly gluten-free as they contain a gluten protein called avenin; however, avenin is generally much better tolerated than the gluten proteins found in wheat, rye, or barley for those who are intolerant. Even some people with celiac disease (severe gluten intolerance) can digest oats—but these must be certified "wheat contaminate-free," since oats are often processed in the same factory as wheat products and may become cross-contaminated.

Quinoa—With its origins from the times of the ancient Inca, this South American grain-like seed is gluten-free and contains vitamin B6, manganese, magnesium, iron, calcium, folate, and zinc. Quinoa is also a complete protein, meaning it contains all eight essential amino acids, which is uncommon in the plant kingdom. Quinoa behaves like a grain in cooking and can be substituted for rice or couscous. It comes in a variety of colors—white, red, and black, with white being the mildest in flavor—and it cooks the same way as rice but can take a little longer. As it swells in cooking water, a little white tail pops out. Be sure to rinse the dry quinoa seeds thoroughly before cooking to remove the bitter saponins that coat it, and rinse until the water stops looking like it has soap bubbles. The saponins may give you a stomachache, but mostly it just makes the quinoa taste bitter and unpleasant. Ideally quinoa should be soaked overnight then rinsed before cooking to reduce phytates (to improve mineral availability). In smoothies, white quinoa is used, and is cooked and cooled before use. Portions of cooked quinoa may also be frozen like porridge discussed previously.

Millet—Also a gluten-free, grain-like seed, millet is a source of manganese, magnesium, calcium, zinc, B vitamins, and vitamin E. It is also considered to be easy to digest, easy to cool, and has anti-inflammatory qualities for the body. Similar to quinoa, millet is cooked and cooled before adding to smoothies. Millet is also cooked like rice but takes longer (30–40 minutes until tender). Portions of cooked millet can be frozen like porridge and quinoa as discussed above.

Fruit in Smoothies

Most recipes will include raw fruit, either in fresh or frozen form. Fruit provides water, fiber, vitamins, minerals, antioxidants, color, texture, and flavor! Fruit is an essential component of my smoothie recipes, particularly to provide the predominant source of sweetness and to provide key nutrients such as vitamin C, some B vitamins, beta-carotene, and manganese. Because vitamin C is so easily degraded, particularly by heat, raw fruit (and leafy greens) are very important to provide this immune-boosting and healing nutrient.

Cooked fruit—Some recipes will call for fruit to be cooked as an option, namely apricots or peaches, which even when ripe aren't always as sweet and juicy as is ideal for addition to smoothies. Cooking will soften and sweeten the fruit. Steaming for 5 to 10 minutes is usually sufficient and is the best way to preserve nutrients and flavor. Some of the kiddie recipes call for cooked apples or pears and I suggest steaming once again. Steaming fruit is also a handy way of getting to eat fruit more quickly, particularly if the weather is cool and it may take a while to ripen. Fruits cooked this way are also delicious atop granola, yogurt or porridge, and as snacks, especially for babies and young toddlers, as they are easy to chew. Hence, it is a wise thing to do to steam more fruit than you need for just one smoothie. Please not that all pre-cooked ingredients are used cold in my smoothie recipes.

A Word on Frozen Ingredients

Fruits that you can buy in abundance when in season and cheap are great to freeze to use for variety in subsequent seasons, including berries and mangoes for winter, and pears for summer.

Use of frozen fruits, especially bananas, adds a creamy element to a smoothie. I always have frozen bananas on hand as I will buy a 30-pound box semi-regularly and when perfectly ripe for smoothies (a little riper than perfect for eating, but not banana cake ripe!), I peel them and freeze in ziplock bags. They thaw quickly, so slice with a knife while frozen and quickly add to the smoothie.

Some blenders require a frozen element to be added, as they tend to warm a smoothie if blending for a long time, such as a green smoothie that requires a longer blend time. Warm smoothies are not pleasant, so if your blender does this, use ice cubes in place of some of the liquid component or some frozen fruit or veg in place of fresh.

Conversely, the use of frozen ingredients can make a smoothie very cold, which may be preferred by some, often fine in summer and hot climates, but is usually not pleasant in winter and very cold climates. To remedy this, add some warm water to the smoothie in place of part of the liquid element.

Personally, I adhere to principles of Ayurveda and Traditional Chinese Medicine when it comes to avoiding the consumption of very cold foods and liquids, for the reason of not interfering with our "digestive fire." I find very cold smoothies harder to digest, but others report that icy-cold smoothies are the only way to go for them. Ultimately, please yourself. Do bear in mind that the more frozen ingredients you use, the thicker the smoothie will be—until it melts.

Fats in Smoothies

Fats are an essential addition to your smoothie because of their many purposes. Fats give your smoothies a smooth, creamy texture, they have great flavor, and most important, they are nutritious. For maternal and child health, fats are a vital part of the diet. For more detailed information on fats, see Chapter 2, "Fabulous Fats."

Nuts and seeds—The addition of nuts and seeds to smoothies can be to add bulk or creaminess and/or for their nutritional profile, given they are packed with fiber, minerals, protein, and healthy fats. They can also be used to add specific nutrients to smoothies, such as calcium from almonds, zinc from sunflower and pumpkin seeds, magnesium from cashews, selenium from Brazil nuts, or omega-3 fats from hemp seeds and walnuts. Whole nuts or seeds or either in butter form may be added to smoothies. Nut or seed milks provide the nutrition of the whole nut or seed minus the fiber, so the end result is lighter. Flavors of milks vary from neutral like almond, to strong like pumpkin seeds. For this reason I only list nut milk, namely almond, for its pleasant and neutral taste; nuts and seeds should be used in whole or buttered forms. My recipe for homemade almond milk is on page 12.

Chia seeds—Chia seeds provide a means to significantly thicken a smoothie if used dry, as they expand at least 10 times their size in liquid. If used pre-soaked, they are not so much of a thickener depending on the quantity used. Chia also adds a source of calcium, magnesium, and omega-3 alpha-linolenic acid (ALA), and is a complete protein (contains all essential amino acids). Flavor of chia is neutral. I don't recommend chia for infants, and this is explained in Chapter 6, "Babies and Toddlers."

Soaking Nuts, Seeds, and Grains

Eating nuts, seeds, and grains after they have been soaked in water for a number of hours is more kind to our digestion and improves nutrient availability. This is because the soaking process helps to deactivate substances that are stopping the nut or seed from growing, particularly protease inhibitors (protease is an enzyme that helps break down protein).

Soaking also aids the removal of anti-nutrients like phytates that can interfere with mineral absorption; however, phytates are more of an issue in grain foods. Soaking also makes the nut or seed softer and easier to blend, which is important if you don't have a high-speed blender.

When soaking grain foods for cooking, like rice and quinoa, the addition of an acidifier helps with the removal of phytates such as whey or lemon juice. For nuts and seeds, the addition of salt to the soak water helps with the removal of the enzyme inhibitors.

When soaking these foods, cover the dry ingredient with plenty of filtered water (plus a little salt for nuts and seeds and some acid for grains), soak for approximately 12 hours, drain the soak water, and rinse thoroughly as the substances you are trying to get rid of will be in the water. An exception is oats, which are low in phytate, so disposing of the soak water isn't necessary. Soaking grains will reduce cooking time by around 5 minutes.

When soaking nuts and seeds, some need a longer soak time and others shorter. For macadamias, cashews, pistachios, and pine nuts, 2 to 4 hours is needed. Don't soak cashews for longer than 4 hours because they go bad very quickly. Personally I don't bother soaking these types of nuts. For Brazil nuts, hazelnuts, sunflower seeds, pumpkin seeds, pecans, or walnuts, soak overnight or all day. Almonds I like to soak for 12 to 24 hours. Hemps seeds require no soaking at all!

Unless it's particularly hot weather, it is fine to soak in bowls on your kitchen counter—otherwise do it in the fridge.

For the purpose of recipes in this book, whether you soak your nuts, seeds, and grains is up to you. All stages of maternal health require optimal nutrition; hence, doing the soaking means more nutrients from these foods and better digestion, which in turn will result in better nutrient absorption. However, the process of soaking nuts, seeds, and grains prior to use can be time-consuming, particularly as a parent—so if you don't it's not the end of the world. It is far better that you use these nutritious foods in any form than to not use them at all. Hence, the soaking of nuts and seeds in particular I have listed as "ideal," but optional, for each applicable recipe. Furthermore if you like the look of a recipe but don't have the nut or seed listed, or you can't eat it for allergy reasons or don't like them, feel free to substitute another that is similar, or simply omit it.

•••

Fresh coconut—Fresh coconut flesh adds beneficial fats as previously discussed, and adds fiber, mild flavor, and creaminess and richness to a smoothie. The only coconut flesh I list in recipes is from young drinking coconuts because the flesh is soft and easy to blend.

Eggs—Raw egg for non-vegans, non-pregnant women, and children over the age of 1 is an excellent source of biotin, choline, and omega-3 fatty acids. You can't really tell they are in your smoothie. The white, while rich in protein, is the more potentially allergenic part, can be hard to digest, and in raw form binds to biotin from the yolk, reducing its availability for absorption. The whole egg, including the white, can be used for boosting protein content of your smoothie; however, the yolk is more nutrient dense. Only reputable sources of eggs should be used (organic-/chemical-free and grass-eating free range), they should be fresh, the shell washed, and each egg checked before putting in your smoothie—it should not smell, white should not be watery, and yolk should not break easily. The risk of salmonella from "conventionally farmed" raw eggs is 1 in 30,000, and even lower and likely negligible with ethical eggs.

Supplementary Ingredients in Smoothies

Other ingredients may be added to smoothies to add flavor or texture, but mostly they add a nutritional element, such as:

Protein powders—I don't often use protein powders as I don't enjoy the mouthfeel of them in my smoothies; however, they can be a great way to improve the range of amino acids consumed in your diet, and protein is essential at each meal if you suffer with blood sugar imbalances. There are many on the market with less-than-desirable ingredients like artificial sweeteners, GMOs (genetically modified organisms), fats, thickeners, milk solids, gluten, or soy, which frequently cause bloating and upset stomachs. I recommend plant-based organic protein powders, and my personal choice is Miessence Complete Protein Powder, which has a combination of pea, rice, and sacha inchi—each of these plant foods has an incomplete set of essential amino acids, but combined they are "complete." I can still tell this powder is in my smoothie, but it is not unpleasant, and my hubby also approves and he is a harder sell then I am! I know if I have had a rough night with my daughter being unsettled, extra protein in my morning smoothies helps my brain kick into gear. The only other brand I am aware of that is comparable in quality is Amazonia Raw protein powder.

Probiotics—Capsules, liquids, or powders mix beautifully in a smoothie and are essential for maternal health. Probiotics will be discussed in more detail in subsequent chapters.

Superfood powders—These superfood powders are abundant on the market now, including mesquite, lucuma, acai berry, baobab, maqui berry, and maca. To some these are very familiar but to most they are not; hence, I have not used them in my recipes to ensure listed ingredients are easy to source or you likely have them at home already. The exception is raw cacao, which is more widely available and popular and can easily be substituted for regular cocoa. Cocoa is roasted and raw cacao is not. The raw form is superior nutritionally with a very high antioxidant content in particular.

Vanilla—You will notice that I list vanilla in many of my smoothie recipes. To me vanilla and smoothies are synonymous but I have refrained from putting vanilla in them all! Please ensure good-quality vanilla in the form of fresh whole beans, vanilla extract, or vanilla paste—not artificial vanilla, which is cheap and nasty. Kids will love the flavor of vanilla, too, but be mindful that the whole bean may leave a slight texture to the smoothie that they may fuss about, so scrape the seeds out and use them only in that case. Paste will be alcohol-free, but not the extract. However, the amount of alcohol that ends up in a smoothie is tiny. There is no consensus as to whether extract should be avoided for kids, so you make that call. If in doubt, use vanilla paste or even vanilla powder if you can get it.

Lemon and lime zest—Lemon and lime zest pack a punch of flavor and bring to life fruits like papaya. They also help the liver to remove excess estrogen from the body, which is especially important for fertility. Please source homegrown or organic citrus for the use of peels as they will not be coated in waxes or chemicals to make them shiny, unlike the conventional varieties you get in the grocery store.

Cinnamon—Such a gorgeous and versatile spice for both sweet and savory foods, cinnamon is very familiar to most people. However, what many don't know is that cinnamon is an umbrella term to describe similar spices harvested from the bark of different plants. True cinnamon is also known as Sri Lankan cinnamon (or Ceylon cinnamon, *Cinnamomum verum*, or *Cinnamomum zeylanicum*), whereas other varieties are actually cassia. The importance of seeking out true cinnamon is that the levels of a substance called coumarin are much lower. Coumarin can be problematic for the liver and is considered too high in quantities less than a teaspoon for an adult and much less than that for kids. A clue that you are eating cassia and not true cinnamon may be irritation of the mucous membranes in the mouth and rash around the mouth—particularly in infants. Ultimately, the best thing to do is to only buy cinnamon that is labeled as Sri Lankan or Ceylon cinnamon. It is not difficult to get, it simply relies on adequate information on the label of the cinnamon you buy. Once you have the good stuff, it not only adds flavor to smoothies but also assists in blood sugar regulation, which is important for hormone balance, mood, and general health.

Turmeric—This spice is well known as an ingredient in Indian curries, but it also works very well in sweet smoothies! Turmeric contains curcumin, which is a powerful antioxidant and is anti-inflammatory in nature. Thanks to these properties, turmeric is considered beneficial for the liver and is very important for hormone health, plus it benefits the joints, cardiovascular system, and brain. Turmeric may be used in powder form and will be characteristically bright yellow. Or during the spring it will be in season in the fresh-root form. Looking a little like ginger but smaller, fresh turmeric is yellow-orange when you cut the flesh; and like the powder, it can stain, so be careful handling it with bare hands and getting it on clothing. For this reason I haven't put any turmeric in baby and toddler smoothies. For simplicity I have only listed turmeric powder, though if you can source it and wish to use the fresh stuff, use 2 to 3 times the volume of fresh to dry. It is also said that the use of black pepper massively enhances the medicinal effects of turmeric. Hence, a grind or two of fresh black pepper could be added to smoothie recipes containing turmeric, but I haven't listed this option. Consider it something you can experiment with if you wish.

Cardamom, cloves, and nutmeg—These lovely spices offer flavor and a hint of warmth to a smoothie. All are antioxidant rich, though the tiny amounts used in smoothies will not be medicinal.

Ginger—Also adding lovely warmth to foods is ginger, which is great added to smoothies, without altering the temperature of the smoothie. Ginger also adds a definite "zing" of flavor. Ginger, like turmeric, is anti-inflammatory and is well known to ease nausea (particularly for motion sickness and morning sickness during pregnancy). It is excellent for the immune system and it is also considered a digestive aid; however, consuming too much can upset the digestive tract.

Smoothie Toppings

It has recently become rather fashionable to place edible items atop smoothies, such as dried coconut, cacao nibs, goji berries, nuts or seeds, whole berries, granola, etc. Toppings make smoothies more interesting to photograph and present nicely in a café setting, particularly atop smoothie bowls. What most people love about smoothies is the simplicity and convenience of them. Eating them with a spoon or spending time decorating the top just complicates matters. If you have the time and the inclination to decorate your smoothies, please go right ahead, but my recipes are just straight-up smoothies (except for the occasional recipes that have passion fruit or pomegranate seeds stirred through them by hand).

Natural Sweeteners

Smoothies, as a general rule, are sweet, and this is the key feature that makes them yummy! Non-green smoothies usually taste great without any added sweetener when sweet fruit is used, such as bananas, mangoes, or melons. Added sweetener will be needed if the ingredients used are sour, such as natural yogurt, lemons, limes, and some berries, or if only small amounts of fruit are used. To make a green smoothie delicious, it is necessary to balance bitterness from the greens and potential fruit or yogurt sourness with sweetness. Ideally, sweet fruit supplies this flavor but sometimes it's not enough. Natural sweeteners used sparingly are the solution and there are numerous options.

Agave nectar—Extracted from the Mexican agave cactus, this sweet and inulin-rich syrup has a low glycemic index (GI) due to the high ratio of fructose it contains compared to glucose. Fructose is metabolized slowly by the liver, versus glucose that is metabolized relatively quickly by all cells in the body. Inulin is a fructan (a chain of fructose molecules) that has beneficial effects on gut flora due to its role as a prebiotic. Look out for organic agave that has had only low heat applied in the production process. Some agave products are highly processed and offer little more nutritionally than high fructose corn syrup, but are even higher in fructose (at around 90 percent). The better quality agave is still around 70 percent fructose. In smoothies, agave imparts a neutral flavor so it's good for "just sweetening." Agave is not suited to those with fructose/fructan malabsorption in particular because it contains both.

Blackstrap molasses—Made from the third boiling of cane sugar syrup, molasses is low in sugar (as sugar crystals are removed in the boiling process) and is a good source of calcium, iron, magnesium, and potassium. As the name suggests it is black in color and robust in flavor. It has roughly equal proportions of glucose and fructose, has a low GI of 55, and is not as sweet as "sugar." Keep in mind that its taste is very strong.

Coconut sugar—This caramel-flavored sugar has a low GI of 35, is considered the most sustainable sweetener in the world to grow, and is a good source of iron, magnesium, and zinc. Made from the sap of the coconut palm blossoms, it is widely available in granulated forms and also as a nectar that the sugar is made from. Coconut sugar is around 48 percent fructose, which is similar to the amount of fructose in regular sugar, and may be tolerated by someone with fructose malabsorption, as glucose and fructose are relatively balanced. Like agave, coconut sugar doesn't influence flavor a great deal in smoothies.

Dates—A fruit with ancient origins, dates are sweet, fibrous, and versatile in the kitchen. Fresh medjool dates are the best option for smoothies because they are soft and blend well. Dates are very sweet and not as nutritious as the dried fruits listed below, but they are a good source of potassium and contain small amounts of a wide variety of vitamins and minerals. Like prunes, dates are sweet but rich in fiber, which slows down the absorption of glucose from them and does not spike blood sugar—hence, they are recommended as a healthy snack for diabetics. If dates are a bit old or have been exposed to the air, they will go a bit dry and will need a soak in water to help them blend better. Due to the high fiber, you may get "bits" in your smoothie if you don't blend very long or don't have a high-powered blender.

Dried fruits—Most well-known dried fruits are apricots, figs, plums (prunes), and raisins, which are concentrated sources of fruity sweetness. But any fruit can be dried, with options such as apples, berries, mangoes, and peaches available commercially. Fruits can also be dried at home using a food dehydrator, which is your best guarantee that your dried fruit doesn't contain preservatives such as the highly allergenic sulfur dioxide (E220), nor coated in "vegetable" oils, which apart from being unnecessary, are either likely to be genetically modified or unethically sourced.

Better options nutritionally are apricots, figs, peaches, and prunes, which are good sources of vitamins A and K, and the minerals calcium, iron, potassium, magnesium, and manganese. Prunes and figs are also a source of B vitamins, particularly B6. Compared to dates, prunes have almost half the sugar, are lower in calories, and more nutritious. Apart from prunes, which are moist, dried fruits should be soaked overnight before use in smoothies, making them easier to blend and avoiding the plumping up effect in the gut that can be dehydrating. Dried fruits are not suitable for those avoiding fructose.

Honey—Apart from dried fruits and dates, honey is the choice for those seeking a sweetener with little to no processing—provided it's unheated and unfiltered. Pure floral honey is the sustaining food source for bees, and contains small amounts of many vitamins, minerals, antioxidants, pollens, and propolis. Regular consumption of raw honey from your local area is thought to assist with controlling seasonal allergies.

Due to its variability, fructose content is reported to range from 36 to 50 percent and hence GI varies too, from 35 to 73, making some honeys, especially Australian bush honeys, low GI (GI below 55). Like agave and coconut sugar, honey (unless it's a strong-tasting bush honey) generally sweetens without imparting much flavor to a smoothie.

Honey is not suitable for strict vegans, and is not to be given to children under 1 year old due to the risk of consuming the botulism toxin. Though very rare, the toxin is more likely in the United States, though after 12 months of age the gut is reported able to handle any ingested spores. Spores are not killed with heat-treated honey. Honey is a wonderfully variable syrup, with looks and tastes that depend on where it's from and what plants the bees visited.

Maple syrup—Sourced from red and black maple trees of North America, this delicious syrup is made by extracting the sap from the trees and thickening it via heating and evaporation. The dark golden liquid must have at least 66 percent sugar and its sugars are mostly made up of sucrose (50:50 glucose:fructose), making maple syrup relatively low in fructose compared to other sweeteners listed here, and it has a GI of 54, which is considered in the low range. Maple syrup has fewer vitamins, but more minerals than honey, namely calcium, iron, manganese, and zinc. Grade B maple syrup, which is harvested later in the season compared to grade A, has a rich, distinctive flavor that can be used to its advantage in smoothies. Grade B is darker, thicker, and has more minerals than grade A. Lighter in color and flow, grade A syrup is better suited for smoothies when maple is the preferred sweetener and flavor imparted needs to be more subtle.

Rice (malt) syrup—Made by culturing brown rice with enzymes to break down the starches, followed by cooking down to syrup, a small amount of glucose and mostly maltose is in the final product. It is completely free of fructose and hence is the preferred sweetener for those avoiding fructose, such as those with fructose malabsorption or on low FODMAP diets for irritable bowl syndrome. Rice malt syrup is gluten-free, suitable for vegans, and has a slow, 90-minute digestion time so it won't spike blood sugar. It is much less sweet than the other sweeteners listed here and won't flavor a smoothie.

Stevia—With leaves 250 times sweeter than sugar and zero calories, stevia is the best option for avoiding processed or unprocessed forms of sugar, such as those listed above. Available in leaf, powder, or tablet forms, stevia doesn't taste as pleasant as other natural sweeteners. To many, including myself, stevia tastes similar to artificial sweeteners such as saccharine. Some commercial preparations of stevia come combined with sugar alcohols, such as erythritol, which makes them taste better and more user-friendly in drinks and cooking due to increased volume. Stevia in the white pill or powdered forms, like sugar alcohols (others are xylitol and sorbitol) are quite processed, which is unattractive to whole-food enthusiasts. Hence, the whole or powdered leaves that are green are the ones to use—but use a little at a time with caution as it's easy to use too much and will ruin your smoothie.

CHAPTER 2

Fabulous Fats

While carbohydrate, protein, and fat are all important and essential macronutrients, fats are particularly essential to all things maternal and fraternal, from preconception through to feeding your children. I am of course talking about good fats. But herein lies a problem: Whose definition of good fats do we believe? That "saturated fats are bad and polyunsaturated fats are good"? Or the opposite? Or is it both? And how about trans fats? To understand why particular fats are considered good or bad, let's take a look at what these fats are.

A fat molecule or "fatty acid" is a group of connected carbon, oxygen, and hydrogen atoms. A fat can be classified according to how long its molecule is and also how "saturated" it is. A medium-chain fat has 6 to 12 carbon atoms at the center of the chain; a long-chain fat has more than 12. If there is just one unsaturated segment (double bonds between carbon atoms), the fat is "monounsaturated," and for multiple segments it's "polyunsaturated." When the bonds are all single, the fat is saturated.

For cellular health, our brains and hormones, we need cholesterol, saturated fats, monounsaturated fats, and poly-unsaturated fats. The human body's fat is 97 percent saturated and monounsaturated, 1.5 percent is omega-3, and 1.5 percent is the rest.

Saturated Fats

Saturated fats are found in plants and animals. The composition of saturated fat means it oxidizes slowly, which makes it a stable, solid fat at room temperature. As a result, it has a great mouthfeel and is great to cook with. In the old days (before omega-6-rich plant oils took over) they were used in most processed foods and baked goods that contained fats (e.g., lard and butter), and were used for deep-frying, such as fish and chips fried in beef tallow.

Saturated medium-chain fats—Coconut, palm (oil) kernels. Their short length allows them to be absorbed directly and they are used as an efficient energy source that doesn't promote weight gain.

Saturated long-chain fats—Animal fats such as butter, cream, lard, and tallow.

Monounsaturated Fats

Monounsaturated fats are long chains and also known as omega-9 fats or oleic acid, which exists in plant foods such as olive, avocado, macadamia, and high-oleic sunflower oil. (Sunflower oil is usually high in omega-6 but there is a high-oleic variety.)

Polyunsaturated Fats

Omega-3 and -6 are long-chain, polyunsaturated fats, also called polyunsaturated fatty acids (PUFAs). We don't need lots of them like we do saturated and monounsaturated fats, but they are a very important component of cell walls, and they influence levels of inflammation in the body, impacting just about everything, especially the health of organs, including the eyes, brain, and heart, plus reproductive organs.

OMEGA-3

Omega-3 from plants is ALA, while omega-3 EPA and DHA are found in microalgae, wild seafood, liver, and to a lesser extent, flesh from animals raised on pasture. The most important is DHA, and the richest source of it is seafood, particularly oily fish. Fish get DHA from eating microalgae such as marine phytoplankton. Land animals, like humans, are not great at converting plant-based ALA that they eat into the longer-chain EPA and DHA, particularly DHA. The ability to convert is dependent upon specific gene expression, gender, and age (greater with younger women), smoking status (worsens), and also dependent on the ratio of LA to ALA being consumed, with too high consumption of LA (linolenic acid) negatively affecting conversion. The key omega-3 fats are:

- ALA (alpha-linolenic acid) found in plants such as seeds and leafy greens.
- EPA (eicosa-pentaenoic acid) found in seafood and algae.
- DHA (docosa-hexaenoic acid) found in seafood, algae, and pastured animal products.

OMEGA-6

The human body is made up of less than 1.5 percent omega-6 fats; yet omega-6 fats are frequently the predominant fat humans are consuming. It is estimated that omega-6 consumption is 10 to 20 times higher than omega-3 in the general population. The ratio of omega-3 to omega-6 fats should be 1:1 to 1:3. But rather than going crazy trying to increase omega-3, such as taking 50 million fish oil capsules daily, it's more sensible to consume more omega-3-rich foods *and* to reduce omega-6 consumption. This means significantly minimizing oils such as canola, safflower, low-oleic sunflower (regular varieties of sunflower oil are low oleic), cottonseed, soy, rice bran, sesame, peanut, and grapeseed. This is easier said than done unless you eat absolutely nothing that comes pre-made—because packaged foods, even relatively healthy ones, are full of vegetable oils instead of saturated animal fats like in the old days. The key omega-6 fats are:

- GLA (gamma-linolenic acid) found in some seeds, greens, and algae.

- LA (linoleic acid) found in nuts and seeds, as well as grain-fed animal products.

- AA (arachidonic acid) found in peanuts and animal products.

Trans Fats

In contrast to saturated fats, the structure of unsaturated fats is unstable. Being liquid at room temperature, they are quicker to oxidize/turn rancid, and hence not as versatile as saturated fats. For this reason, the food technology industry developed the process of "hydrogenation," which creates a partially saturated fat, from an unsaturated fat, to produce "foods" such as margarine or vegetable shortening that are no longer liquid fats and have a long shelf life. This process produces trans fats, which have an altered molecular structure that is complex and full of nasty chemicals. Trans fats in recent years have been removed from the end product of things like margarine, but this is still not a good fat in any way, having no nutritional value in its altered state.

Synthetically altered fats confuse the body and are integrated into cell walls, upsetting the balance of saturated fats, cholesterol, and omega-3 and -6 fats that ensure the cell wall functions optimally to transport nutrients in and waste out. If this process isn't working, it contributes to inflammation and illness with a cell wall that is too rigid. An imbalance of PUFAs can be problematic, too, for similar reasons, as omega-3 creates flexibility while omega-6 makes the walls more rigid.

Every major health organization in the world agrees trans fats are bad and omega-3 oils are good. But unfortunately, the vast majority of the world believes saturated fats and cholesterol are bad and omega-6 vegetable oils are good. Thankfully, the latter is slowly losing traction, as it's the consumption of too much sugar, trans fats, and too much omega-6 linoleic acid (LA) that results in inflammation that damages blood vessel walls, leading to cardiovascular disease. I highly recommend you read *Toxic Oil* by David Gillespie for a more detailed analysis of fats.

Cholesterol

Cholesterol is essential to the makeup of our cell membranes and an important precursor to steroid hormones (such as progesterone and testosterone), bile salts (which help us digest fat), and vitamin D. Cholesterol is therefore pretty important for maternal health, and for fertility for men and women. Cholesterol is found in the fats from animal products, and in the human body it is transported within the structure of "lipoproteins." Low-density lipoproteins (LDL) transport fats in the blood to cells where they are needed, and high-density lipoproteins (HDL) carry unused fats back to the liver.

Between 60 and 80 percent of cholesterol is in LDL and is considered in mainstream medicine to be the "bad" cholesterol, with HDL being good. The thing is, neither is good nor bad, they simply both exist to perform a job and both are equally important. What is "bad" is when LDL becomes oxidized, which occurs when LDL transports polyunsaturated omega-6 fats (namely LA) rather than monounsaturated and saturated fats. LA from nut, grain, and seed oils is more prone to structural damage by oxygen and in turn free radicals are created; then in the absence of enough antioxidants to neutralize them, "oxidized LDL" is formed, which is associated with heart disease, unlike healthy LDL, which isn't.

Hence, it is important to consume saturated and mono-unsaturated fats and limit omega-6 LA to assist with healthy LDL levels. LDL transporting our "good fats" results in the delivery of the right fats to the right places and this will contribute to hormone balance—essential for maternal and paternal health.

Fats and Fertility

With regard to fertility, omega-3 fats have a blood-thinning effect, and hence improve blood flow to organs such as the brain, heart, and reproductive organs. Good blood flow to the uterus and ovaries in women, and genitals in men, means improved fertility with support to hormone production and function of the ovaries and testes to release eggs and sperm, respectively. Reduction of blood pressure and depressive symptoms in men may also help issues with erectile dysfunction. In women, omega-3 fats help to increase the egg-white-like mucus during the time of ovulation, which is needed to help mobilize sperm toward the egg. Omega-3 DHA is also an essential part of a mature sperm's outer membrane, which helps create healthy and motile swimmers!

Fats, especially saturated fats and cholesterol, are essential for making hormones, which explains why women (and men) who are on low-fat diets and are too lean, or who have very low cholesterol levels, are more likely to be infertile due to inadequate hormone production, especially progesterone in women and testosterone in men. The exception to avoiding excessive omega-6 is GLA, which is anti-inflammatory in nature and excellent for the premenstrual stage in particular.

Nuts and Seeds

It's important not to go overboard eating nuts and seeds as they are, for the most part, rich sources of omega-6 LA (except macadamia, chia, and flax). Nuts and seeds, however, are not concentrated oils—they also contain protein, carbohydrate, and fiber, and are far better to consume whole than the oils that are made from them. Apart from macadamias, which are around 60 percent fat by weight, other nuts and seeds are less than 50 percent fat by weight, compared to any oil, which is 100 percent fat.

Hemp seeds and walnuts are both good sources of omega-3 ALA but have more omega-6 than -3. Hemp has the ratio of 3:1 and walnuts 4.3:1. Sunflower seeds, which don't contain much omega-3, do have a 3:1 ratio of omega-6:3, which is better than the 11:1 that pumpkin seeds have. Apart from macadamias, which have very little omega-3 or -6 fats, the other listed nuts, eggs, and avocado will still contribute to omega-6 load. Other nuts such as cashews and Brazils are still beneficial for nutritional reasons, eaten whole, as butters, or for making milks. Just bear in mind they are all sources of omega-6, which needs to be considered in relation to the rest of the diet. If vegetable oils are otherwise kept to a minimum and copious amounts of nuts and seeds aren't being eaten—big handfuls—then modest additions to smoothies are not a big problem.

Fats during Pregnancy and Breastfeeding

The most important omega-3 fat during pregnancy is DHA, which is essential to babies' brain, eye, and nervous system development. DHA represents over 90 percent of all omega-3 fats in the brain, and in the retina of the eye. The importance of DHA to the central nervous system extends from pregnancy and up to 18 months of a child's life. During the third trimester of pregnancy, the fetus's brain growth is at its peak, with the fetus's highest need for DHA at 50mg to 70mg a day. Babies must obtain DHA via the placenta during pregnancy, from breast milk (or fortified formula) following birth, and from milk and food after around 6 months of age. DHA is also important for maternal well-being via improvement to mood, and adequate DHA assists babies to be carried to term.

Omega-6 AA (arachidonic acid) can be supplied by the diet, namely from animal products especially chicken and eggs. It can also be synthesized in the body from the supply of LA (which is rarely in short supply). It is critical to the development of the fetal and infant central nervous system with DHA, and AA is part of all cell membranes in the body with EPA. Because AA is a precursor to series 2 prostaglandins (PG2) and thromboxane, we don't want too much—they are associated with preterm labor and preeclampsia, respectively. However, it is the PG2 that is used to induce labor when it's required. Adequate supply of both omega-3 DHA and EPA helps to keep AA levels under control. In contrast EPA is a precursor to series 3 prostaglandins, which help to keep the muscular middle layer of the uterus relaxed. EPA is also believed to be important to control the movement of both DHA and AA across the placenta.

Low levels of DHA predispose breastfeeding mothers to poor mood, stress intolerance, and increased risk for postpartum depression, because DHA will be preferentially transferred to the baby in utero and through her breast milk, leaving the mother deficient. DHA entering breast milk is also dependent on the mother's diet. Coconut oil, zinc, iron, and vitamin B6 assist the conversion of plant-based ALA to DHA, but the conversion can be as little as 0.5 percent. In women of childbearing years, estrogens can increase this conversion to around 20 percent, which is pretty darn clever given the extra need! However, it is still wise to take a DHA supplement while pregnant and breastfeeding.

Deficiency of DHA pre- and postnatally can implicate problems with a child's learning and behavior for life. Furthermore, deficiency from generation to generation sees these problems escalate, which is what is being observed in recent decades, as Western diets provide insufficient DHA (less than 100mg) and are overly abundant in omega-6 plant oils. The primary dietary sources of DHA are oily fish and liver—neither of which is commonplace in a typical Western diet, and both of which pregnant women are advised to limit for risk of ingesting toxins such as mercury and too much vitamin A, respectively. Subsequently, experts worldwide recommend supplementing at 200mg to 300mg of DHA daily while pregnant and breastfeeding, and up to 1,000mg according to some sources. I was prescribed DHA at this much higher dose. Do note that most fish oil supplements have a higher ratio of EPA to DHA, so seek out ones that are high in DHA and still contain some EPA.

Importance of Fat for Nutrient Absorption

In addition to the specific important roles fats play in women's and men's health, fats are also required to aid nutrient absorption for everyone—and in times of extra demand for nutrients such as pregnancy and lactation, this is even more important. The fat-soluble vitamins A, D, E, and K require fat as a carrier to be absorbed by the body. Because fat-soluble vitamins can be stored in the liver and fatty body tissues, they don't need to be supplied daily. When consuming these vitamins, it's important that if they don't come packaged with some fat already, such as avocadoes, nuts, eggs, etc., they need to be consumed with added fat. This is one reason why it's important that milks are not low fat or fat free, especially dairy milk, and it's important to add fat to a salad, such as olives, avocado, and/or a dressing with oil. Similarly, adding fat like coconut oil or butter to steamed veggies is beneficial, and of course putting some fat in a smoothie helps—even just a little bit. With regard to heat being applied to foods, fat-soluble vitamins, like minerals, are preserved when heated, unlike vitamins C and B5, which are easily damaged by heat, and folate, which is denatured at around 140°F (60°C) and B1 at greater than 212°F (100°C). Hence these latter nutrients should ideally be consumed raw and unheated.

Where to Get Your Oils

For preconception, pregnancy, and breastfeeding, DHA needs to be consumed from the foods it exists in and/or from supplementation. What is also required is not just to eat more omega-3 oils but also to reduce omega-6 oils, and to balance omega-3 ALA relatively equally with omega-6 LA from plant sources.

Omega-6 is present in nut, seed, legume, and grain oils. Foods that boast omega-3 also contain omega-6, and often in a greater ratio, such as in eggs, hemp, and walnuts. The best sources of omega-3 without omega-6 dominance are oily fish, flax, and chia. Let's refrain from making fishy smoothies, however! And we will stick to using flax or chia (chia is preferred due to its neutral taste and it's easier to blend) when we want an omega-3 boost. It's still okay to use eggs, hemp, walnuts, and other nuts and seeds, as they are still beneficial to our health for other reasons such as minerals and protein, as long as your diet overall is not omega-6 dominant, with foods cooked in vegetable oils, animals raised on grains not pasture, and if it does not contain a lot of grains. Animals raised on pasture have higher omega-3 in their tissues than when fed omega-3-rich feed and not pastured; however, it should be noted that there is more ALA in plants than pastured meat, and more omega-3 EPA and DHA in seafood than pastured meat.

The omega-6 oil that is an exception is GLA, which is anti-inflammatory in nature and can be found in the seeds of borage, black currant and evening primrose, to a lesser extent in hemp and olive oils, and in the microalgae spirulina. GLA and DHA are found in breast milk and are dependent upon the mother's diet.

Coconuts

Coconuts are such an amazing and versatile food with oil, butter, water, milk, cream, fresh or dried flesh (shredded, flakes, desiccated), and flour all available from the one superb orb! In Sanskrit, the coconut palm is known as *kalpa vrisksha* or "the tree that supplies all that is needed to live." Coconut has 47 percent lauric acid, which is the fat in mother's milk that makes it so special. It aids digestion and absorption of minerals and fat-soluble vitamins, is good for blood sugar, and is antifungal, antiviral, and antibacterial; hence, it's great for the immune system. I use coconut products frequently in my smoothies and everyday foods. Coconut products that suit smoothies the best include the milk, cream, and the fresh flesh and water from "drinking" coconuts (also known as Thai, young, or green coconuts).

Coconut oil is a saturated fat, which refers to its structure having all possible links to it filled with hydrogen atoms. Unlike the long-chain saturated fats from animal products, coconut oil is a medium-chain fat. Because it is shorter, it is metabolized by the body quickly and efficiently into energy; hence it can aid weight loss via its metabolism-boosting and thyroid-nourishing qualities. It is also rich in antioxidants so it makes the oil very stable, unlike flax oil that can rapidly go rancid, nor like other plant oils that will go rancid slowly.

To be added successfully to smoothies, coconut oil needs to be soft or runny so its blends well. However, this will only work if the other ingredients are not cold, because coconut oil solidifies below 64°F (18°C), above 79°F (26°C) it will turn to liquid, and its buttery in between. For the same reason, it won't work as liquefied oil in a dressing or over salad, as it will go hard on the cool food. So while coconut oil can be put in a smoothie, it's a bit temperamental and I have chosen not to use it in my recipes. Coconut oil is, however, excellent for cooking, especially for curries and stir-fries. It can be used instead of butter in baking, stirred through warm quinoa or rice, or melted on steamed veggies. Coconut oil is also great as a body lotion, is used for dental health via oil pulling, and is an excellent all-natural lubricant in the bedroom! Be sure to buy organic, cold-pressed coconut oil to ensure quality and no chemical contamination. Some are quite strong in smell and flavor and others mild.

The fresh flesh of a drinking coconut may be jelly-like or be firm, but not hard like a mature coconut. You can put the flesh straight into a smoothie, simply eat it as is, slice it into noodles for salads and stir-fries, make coconut ice cream, coconut yogurt—the list goes on! The flesh will last a few days in the fridge and also freezes well. When jelly-like, the flesh will impart a lovely silkiness to your smoothie. When firmer, it will provide more fiber and a little texture, but is still delicious.

Fresh coconut water contains a balance of electrolytes, including sodium, potassium, calcium, and magnesium—so beneficial that it was used in old war times as an emergency replacement for blood plasma! It is delicately sweet and makes a beautiful and very healthy base to a smoothie, particularly green smoothies, as the sweetness helps to balance the bitterness of the greenery used. Coconut water is easily bought commercially these days, but it is expensive, doesn't taste as good as fresh, and some brands use heat in its processing and use preservatives for packaging. So it's better to use preservative-free, unsweetened, and raw (non-heat treated) coconut water brands. How to access the water and flesh from a fresh coconut is explained below.

HOW TO OPEN A DRINKING COCONUT

After the husk is shaved off for the purpose of sales in grocery stores, drinking coconuts look cylindrical and white, with a pointed top and a flat bottom, versus a mature coconut that is round, brown, and hairy looking. Opening a drinking coconut is a challenge when first confronted with one and there are different successful methods. Ultimately, you want a hole in the top to pour out the liquid and a hole large enough to scoop out the flesh. Initially I would use the heel of a big knife to whack down hard on about five points of the top without shaving any of the top off. It worked, though it does result in bits of coconut husk and coconut water flying around, which is not so good in the kitchen! My dad used a large drill bit for a while, which was rather novel, though perhaps not hygienic. Others do it with a very sharp cleaver: four whacks in a square and it's open—rather scary but quick and effective! The following, however, is the safe and very simple method I use now:

- Turn the coconut on its side. With a large, sturdy kitchen knife, shave the white husk off the pointed end, down to the pale brown shell.

- Turn the coconut up onto its base again. On the top there are three naturally occurring thick lines that meet at the apex. With the heel of the same knife, tap firmly on one of these lines about halfway along till it cracks the shell—not much force is needed.

- Stick the heel of the knife in the crack, and with a bit of leverage you will create a continuation of the crack in a perfect circle around the top that you can pry open.

- Empty the water into a bowl over a fine sieve to catch any debris, and check that the water is a clear/white color. If it's pink, purple or brown, or it doesn't taste amazing, throw it out! It is unfortunately not uncommon for drinking coconuts to have rancid water.

- To scoop out the flesh, use the back of a soup spoon to scrape the flesh off the shell. You should almost be able to remove it in one piece if it's thick enough. Rinse under water and scrape off any brown bits from the shell.

- To see photos or a video of this process please visit www .kristinemiles.com.

A Summary of Fats

The best sources of recommended smoothie-friendly good fats to consume are:

- Saturated: coconut (fresh flesh from drinking coconuts, milk, cream), raw eggs
- Monounsaturated (oleic/omega-9): avocado, macadamias, sunflower seeds, almonds, pecans, walnuts
- Polyunsaturated omega-3 ALA: chia, flax, hemp, walnuts
- Polyunsaturated GLA: hemp
- Cholesterol: raw eggs

DHA and EPA are not something you can get a lot of in smoothies, particularly when raw eggs in smoothies are out during pregnancy and won't be given to babies, but smoothies are not going to be the only thing you consume, so be sure to get DHA and EPA from other sources in your diet, plus a good-quality DHA supplement.

CHAPTER 3

Making Babies

So you've decided to make a baby! How wonderful! If it's your first, you are on an amazing journey of education and discovery. If it's a subsequent child you're planning, then you've already experienced and learned so much. If you're reading this chapter and you are pregnant already, then congratulations! Please keep reading because many of the principles of preconception care are relevant to pregnancy, namely optimizing nutrition for the benefit of you and your child.

The idea of preconception care can have variable meaning. For some it's simply focusing on the task at hand and planning when in the month to have intercourse. For others it's an all-encompassing physical, emotional, and medical journey toward holding their precious bundle in their arms. Some couples become pregnant quite easily on their first or second attempt, but many don't. And on top of that, half of pregnancies are unplanned.

Taking time to prepare for conception is a valuable thing to do. It takes 4 months for a female egg to mature and sperm to form.

The difference between a healthy, well-formed egg and sperm in addition to well-balanced hormones can mean the difference between becoming and staying pregnant easily or not. It can influence the quality of the pregnancy, as well as the growth and health of the baby. Whether you are just starting out trying to conceive, thinking about it, or experiencing infertility, it is equally important to prepare your body and that of your partner. Unlike pregnancy and breastfeeding, which have all the focus on the mother's nutrition and well-being, conception responsibilities must be equally shared between mother and father. This includes aiming for a natural conception, or the use of assisted reproductive technologies such as in vitro fertilization (IVF). Therefore, abstaining from alcohol and optimizing nutrition and well-being need to be by *both parents*, because hormone imbalances not only affect a woman's menstrual cycle, they affect a man's sperm production and quality too.

While it's ideal to prepare at least 4 months in advance, if you have fallen pregnant easily already then fantastic! If, however, you have been trying to get pregnant and it's not happening, then having a break and undertaking preconception care is an option (in combination with further investigation). This is something I did. After 3 years of "trying," nothing was happening. I had been medically investigated, including exploratory surgery and lots of blood tests, and no explanation was found, nor was preconception preparation even mentioned. I subsequently started a program with a natural fertility specialist, which included many more tests and finally some answers. I committed to a 4-month preconception program over which time my hormones rebalanced, and we became pregnant on our second month trying afterward.

GABRIELA ROSA'S STORY

Before even thinking of conception, I ensured I followed my own Fertility Alignment Program. I made sure both my husband and I were as healthy as possible prior to our conception attempts. It's safe to say we followed my own advice of "act pregnant now to get pregnant later" to a tee as a couple. We led a very healthy lifestyle, essentially everything I ask of my patients. This was quite important because my husband's sperm was quite below par with 0 percent morphology some years before, and because of my polycystic ovary syndrome (PCOS), treatment was even more important because I had come from having one period a year to a regular cycle. It was quite a lot of "work." The good news is that it truly paid handsomely with a healthy baby conceived, first try. —Gabriela

Nutrients Recommended for Prenatal Women and Men

Nutrition plays a very important role with fertility—namely for hormone health and the formation and function of egg and sperm. It's not the only important factor when it comes to fertility, but given this book is all about smoothies, then we are interested in smoothie- and conception-friendly ingredients.

MICRONUTRIENTS

Folate

Folic acid is probably the most famous recommended prenatal nutrient. The term folic acid is frequently used interchangeably with folate, but it is actually the synthetic form, which is in most supplements, and folate (or vitamin B9) is the natural form in plants (and liver). First recognized in 1970 as a necessary nutrient to help prevent neural tube birth defects, it wasn't an official recommendation to take 400mcg for women of childbearing age until 1992, and fortification in foods began in 1998. This is because standard diets tend to only provide around 200mcg, and 40 to 50 percent of pregnancies are believed to be unplanned. Depending on the source, it is advised to take up to 1200mcg per day when planning to get pregnant, but usually it's between 400mcg and 800mcg.

Folate is needed to make healthy new cells, and given there is a lot of cell division going on when a fetus is developing in the first 3 months of gestation, it is essential! Specifically, it is marketed to prevent spina bifida, which occurs in utero where the baby's spinal column does not close over to protect the spinal cord, which can lead to lifelong disability; or anencephaly, which is fatal, where part of the brain, skull, and scalp are missing. With a history of you or a family member having a baby with a brain or spine defect, it may be professionally recommended to take 4000mcg, which cannot be met by diet alone.

Folate is also needed for male fertility for sperm quality and in similar levels to women. Better quality sperm means a better chance of hitting the target—that is, the egg—and lessens the chance of abnormal sperm fertilizing an egg and potentially causing birth defects.

Folate is metabolized well in the lining of the small intestine and can cross the placenta to be delivered to a growing baby—folic acid does not. Folic acid must go through a complex series of reactions to be in a usable form, which requires specific enzymes and nutrients such as serine, glycine, vitamins B12, B2, and B6. If any of these nutrients is lacking, you have a problem. Moreover, if you have a common genetic mutation (MTHFR) that affects the production of these necessary enzymes, this is also a problem, because it results in unmetabolized folic acid in the blood, which can mask a B12 deficiency, affect immunity, and won't be beneficial in the prevention of neural tube defects. Blood tests may suggest a great level of folic acid in the blood, but it's not where it should be in a form that is useful. What makes this issue nice and confusing is that many sources say that folic acid is better absorbed than folate and promote the use of the synthetic form. Mother Nature designed folate to do the job, not a synthetic version. Hence it is wise to avoid folic acid in supplements and fortified foods, and instead look out for 5-methyltetrahydrofolate or 5-MTHF, L-methylfolate, or Metafolin in supplement form. And of course, a daily green smoothie goes a long way to providing essential folate for parents to be, with around 100mcg in just a 50g serving of spinach alone.

Smoothie- and fertility-friendly sources: leafy greens, especially spinach, collards, kale, parsley and romaine lettuce; avocado, peanuts, beets, oranges, papaya, mangoes, banana, sunflower seeds, walnuts, and cantaloupe

Vitamin B12

This essential nutrient for male and female fertility is a water-soluble vitamin only found in animal products. We only need 1mcg daily, but that tiny little bit is super important for our mood, healthy blood, nervous system, detoxification, and hormone balance. Vitamin B12 contains the trace mineral cobalt, and hence it's other name "cobalamin." Like folate, vitamin B12 is usually supplemented in a synthetic form—cyanocobalamin—which is also poorly utilized if the MTHFR gene mutation is present, as it limits the ability of cyanocobalamin to be converted to methylcobalamin (the usable form in the body). More on MTHFR will be discussed on page 74.

Smoothie- and fertility-friendly sources: raw eggs

Note: In creamy smoothies with banana and/or milk or nuts, you won't even notice eggs in there, but in a watery smoothie such as one based on melon, it won't be very pleasant and isn't recommended.

Magnesium

Magnesium regulates over 300 enzyme reactions in the body. It is particularly important for energy and it relaxes the nervous system. Deficiency can produce symptoms of anxiety, depression, poor sleep, poor memory, muscle weakness and twitches/cramps, and fatigue. Magnesium is also needed for the metabolism of estrogen, and for the synthesis of progesterone with vitamin B6 and zinc. Estrogen is cumulatively higher in the second half of the menstrual cycle (the luteal phase), and progesterone is significantly higher; hence the tendency to have symptoms of magnesium deficiency in the latter part of the cycle, which will contribute to premenstrual symptoms such as cramping, headaches, moodiness, insomnia, and constipation—as well as cravings for chocolate, which is magnesium rich!

Nutritional needs are higher in the luteal phase generally due to the higher hormone activity, and hand in hand with this is the additional need for sleep, plus avoiding toxins and junk food. If your body is under stress and needs to work hard at detoxifying from poor lifestyle choices, then it will use up nutrients that are needed for your hormones at the expense of hormone balance, which not only contributes to premenstrual syndrome (PMS) but also to infertility. Because magnesium is known as "the great relaxer," it is suggested that a deficiency can put the uterus and fallopian tubes in a state of tension and even spasm that can impact implantation of a fertilized egg. Magnesium is also

important for blood sugar control as insulin needs magnesium for
its manufacture and transport.

Smoothie- and fertility-friendly sources: nuts and seeds,
especially pumpkin seeds and tahini; cacao; leafy greens, such
as spinach, mint, beet leaves, Swiss chard, and kale; and beets,
blackberries, raspberries, quinoa, oats, hemp seeds, chia, bananas,
and figs

Selenium

Selenium is a powerful antioxidant and free-radical scavenger,
and works alongside other nutrients that function as antioxidants
or co-factors for antioxidant enzymes, such as zinc, manganese,
and vitamins C and E. Selenium combines with the amino acids
cysteine and methionine to form glutathione peroxidase, which is
essential to protect the liver from damage by peroxides, which find
their way into the body via exposure to chemical-based cleaning
products such as disinfectants, detergents, and bleaches. (Seeking
out natural and chemical-free options for cleaning, cosmetics,
food, and office supplies is an obvious way to reduce the need
for glutathione peroxidase, and hence any significant need for
selenium in the first place.)

With a deficiency of selenium comes oxidative stress. Oxidative
stress means free radicals are generated, and these can cause
damage to the DNA, which can result in the death or damage to
cells anywhere in the body and anywhere in the reproductive area
of men and women. This subsequently influences egg and sperm
production—specifically sperm motility via the production of the
tail, and ultimately egg fertilization and pregnancy. Deficiency is
also linked with the potential complications of miscarriage, low
birth weight babies, premature babies, birth defects, preeclampsia,
and gestational diabetes.

Selenium contributes to testosterone production in men and is also an essential nutrient for the thyroid, exhibiting an anti-inflammatory effect and reducing anti-thyroid antibodies if present. Selenium and zinc are required to convert the thyroid hormone T4 into T3. More information on the thyroid on page 67.

Smoothie- and fertility-friendly sources: Selenium is particularly rich in Brazil nuts and to a lesser extent in eggs, sunflower seeds, cashews, macadamias, and oats.

Zinc

More than 300 biological functions in the human body require zinc, and in particular, zinc is necessary for the synthesis of all proteins in the body including genetic material. Hence it is one of the most important fertility nutrients for men and women, as it directly influences the quality of eggs and sperm. Zinc is important for the immune system, balancing blood sugar, detoxification, healthy skin and hair, and it helps convert beta-carotene to retinol (vitamin A), helps T4 convert to T3, and helps lower homocysteine.

Zinc is also involved in energy metabolism, and the reason sperm contain a high level of zinc is to give them the energy they need to reach the egg and create and release enzymes to help the sperm head to penetrate the egg's outer shell. Zinc also aids sperm motility by preventing them from clumping together, which slows them down.

For women, zinc is important for the immune system, balancing blood sugar, detoxification, and hormone balance because zinc is needed to make progesterone. Hormone imbalance can affect how regular a menstrual cycle is, and how an ovary develops and releases its eggs. Zinc is easily depleted by other minerals such as copper and iron, so if taking iron and zinc supplements, take them at different times of day. Zinc can also be depleted if the diet is high in phytates from grains and is the predominant mineral to be malabsorbed with issues such as gluten intolerance. Zinc is also needed to convert beta-carotene from plants to the active form of vitamin A—another important fertility nutrient.

Smoothie- and fertility-friendly sources: cacao, chia, coconut, cashews, Swiss chard, parsley, eggs, macadamias, maple syrup, oats, pecans, peanuts, hemp seeds, pumpkin seeds, tahini, figs, spinach, ginger root, almonds, and sunflower seeds

Vitamin A

Vitamin A is an antioxidant and fat-soluble vitamin that is important for our immune system, skin, mucous membranes, and eye health. With regard to reproduction, vitamin A is what keeps the fine hair-like structures called "cilia" in the fallopian tubes moving well, to assist the movement of sperm to the egg. Vitamin A works with cholesterol to produce estrogen and testosterone. Like zinc, vitamin A also prevents sperm from clumping together, so it aids motility. Additionally, it improves the quality of fertile cervical mucus, which helps sperm live longer and hence offers more chance of reaching the desired destination!

As described by the Weston A. Price Foundation for Wise Traditions in Food, Farming, and the Healing Arts (westonaprice .org), traditional cultures fed women trying to conceive a diet rich in vitamin A from organ meats (especially liver) and butter from grass-fed cows. A single 100g serving of liver can be over 50,000IU. The worldwide guidelines don't recommend taking more than 10,000IU of vitamin A. Regardless of what is safe or not, it's still best to be guided by your treating health practitioner as to appropriate amounts to take.

Plant and animal sources will always be a safer option than synthetic versions of vitamin A and will be better absorbed and metabolized. Preformed vitamin A (retinol) from animals is more easily assimilated because beta-carotene from plants must be converted to retinol. In fact, one beta-carotene molecule makes two retinol molecules, and the body will do this conversion as needed by utilizing enzymes and zinc in the process. If not enough retinol is being consumed, then beta-carotene will be used to top it up.

Smoothie- and fertility-friendly sources: eggs, carrots, pumpkin, sweet potato, spinach, kale, cantaloupe, mango, papaya, pineapples, passion fruit, apricots, peaches, nectarines, and kiwi

Vitamin C

Vitamin C is well known for its immune-boosting role thanks to its antioxidant and detoxifying properties. It is also essential for collagen formation, which is what our soft tissues are made of, such as muscles, skin, and the connective tissues of our joints.

It is a detoxifying antioxidant nutrient, making it important to help deal with toxins in our bodies that may interfere with hormone balance and formation of healthy cells. Vitamin C also aids the absorption of other nutrients such as the B vitamins, vitamin D, and especially the mineral iron. Vitamin C is in plentiful supply in the ovaries and is necessary for the production sex hormones, particularly progesterone. In men, vitamin C is important for preventing sperm from clumping together.

Vitamin C also complements the action of antioxidant phytochemicals such as bioflavonoids, which are abundant in citrus and tropical fruit, and anthocyanins, which are color pigments found in berries, cherries, grapes, plums, and bananas.

Smoothie- and fertility-friendly sources: brassicas (or cruciferous vegetables), parsley, papaya, avocado, passion fruit, beets, pomegranates, strawberries, mangoes, bananas, kiwi, citrus, and melons

Note: Vitamin C is the most fragile vitamin, being prone to oxidation by heat and air exposure, so to maximize vitamin C availability, eat (or drink) vitamin C–rich foods raw, and consume quickly after preparation.

Vitamin E

Like vitamin C, vitamin E is important for immunity, and strength and healing of our soft tissues. In men, vitamin E is particularly important for sperm count, quality, and motility. Significant vitamin E deficiency is linked with infertility in men through lack of sperm in semen. In women, vitamin E also helps thicken the lining of the uterus. Unlike vitamin C, which is water soluble, vitamin E is a fat-soluble vitamin, meaning it dissolves in fat, and so it needs fat to be absorbed. This is why it's good to have a least a little fat in smoothies, to ensure there is a source of fat for the absorption of fat-soluble vitamins and minerals. Care must be taken with fat-soluble vitamins, as the body does not eliminate them via the urine if there is more than required in the body. They can accumulate in higher than helpful doses and interfere with other bodily functions, and in the case of vitamin E, it can interfere with the function of vitamin K and impact blood clotting. Vitamin E overdosing is unlikely from food sources, and any vitamin or mineral supplementation, particularly fat-soluble nutrients, should be under the guidance of an appropriate health professional.

Smoothie- and fertility-friendly sources: leafy greens (especially chard and spinach), avocado, sunflower seeds, almonds, peanuts, mint, papaya, kiwi, nectarines, and raspberries

Iron

Iron is one of the most infamous nutrients of pregnancy, given it is prone to deficiency due to its very high need. Iron is needed for the formation of red blood cells, which contain hemoglobin, the iron-containing protein that carries oxygen around the body to all tissues—including reproductive organs. Maternal blood volume increases by 50 percent to support a growing baby (and growing mother!), and iron is essential for rapidly growing and differentiating cells. Hence, iron deficiency may be linked to infertility in the form of anovulation (lack of ovulation) or poor egg quality, due to poor oxygen supply to the ovaries, and also interference to cell division leading to miscarriage—which is perhaps an insurance policy in itself, as going into a pregnancy while anemic poses great risk to the development of a baby's blood supply and organ development, especially the brain.

Iron is tested via a number of parameters. Iron or "serum iron" is the amount of iron in the blood. "Ferritin" is a protein that stores iron. Serum iron usually does not fall until ferritin is depleted. Hence, simply testing for iron in the blood may miss a problem with stored iron. Heme iron, which comes from animal sources, is more easily absorbed than non-heme iron found from plants. Vitamin C, sugars, copper, and amino acids assist iron absorption; vitamin A helps release stored iron, and non-heme iron absorption is also improved by the presence of heme iron. Phosphates in eggs, milk, and cheese, as well as oxalic acid, phytic acid, and tannins, decrease absorption, which is why in addition to dairy being low in iron, dairy milk is not recommended as a drink for infants under 1 year old. Caffeinated drinks and some herbal teas such as peppermint and chamomile can also reduce absorption due to their polyphenol content. Zinc and iron tablets taken together inhibit zinc absorption, and iron and calcium taken together inhibit iron absorption.

Confused? Don't panic! Eat a balanced and varied diet rich in vitamin C and A, take zinc and calcium supplements in the evening and iron in the morning (if you happen to be taking these supplements), and avoid drinking teas and coffee with meals—drink between meals or not at all (caffeine isn't optimal for fertility anyway; more on that later)—and iron from your diet should end up where it's needed. If you are anemic and trying to conceive, please get professional advice regarding increasing your ferritin levels, and achieve this *before* you start trying.

Smoothie- and fertility-friendly sources (heme iron): raw eggs

Smoothie- and fertility-friendly sources (non-heme iron): leafy greens, especially spinach, chard, and parsley; dried apricots, figs, raspberries, raisins, prunes, beets, cacao, tahini, turmeric, pumpkin seeds, hemp seeds, chia, and quinoa

....

Oxalates, Phytates, and Tannins

Oxalates, phytates, and tannins can negatively affect absorption of other minerals. Thankfully, there are ways around this without necessarily avoiding the foods they are present in.

OXALATES

Oxalic acid, which is present in many foods (including leafy greens such as spinach, chard, and parsley, as well as some berries, nuts, oats, buckwheat, soy products, quinoa, chocolate, and wheat), can bind with calcium, magnesium, sodium, potassium, or iron to form oxalate minerals. Most of these minerals are water soluble and are excreted through the urine, but calcium oxalate is insoluble, and is found in 80 percent of kidney stones. Some sources would have you believe that the consumption of raw leafy greens is detrimental to your health due to the risk of calcium oxalate forming and thus causing kidney stones. However, it is the reduced consumption of water and high consumption of animal protein, cornstarch, and high fructose corn syrup, and the consumption of inorganic calcium supplements that are relevant to kidney stone formation.

There is no definitive evidence that reducing dietary oxalic acid alters the risk of developing stones. Furthermore, cooking only reduces the oxalic acid content by a small amount, so cooking greens does not make much of a difference. And let's not forget the prevalence of oxalic acids in any everyday foods and not just greens. The epidemiology of calcium oxalate stones suggest middle-aged men are at greater risk—hardly the typical green-smoothie-swilling, health-seeking types. (Apologies to any green-smoothie-loving middle-aged men out there!)

Taking magnesium is recommend to help prevent calcium oxalate stone formation. Hence instead of calcium plus oxalic acid forming calcium oxalate, the presence of magnesium ideally results in the formation of water-soluble magnesium oxalate that is simply peed out. The key preventer, however, appears to be adequate hydration, so that urine isn't too concentrated, which encourages oxalates to form as they are floating closer together to calcium ions. Interestingly, many of the listed foods high in oxalate are also sources of magnesium (and/or calcium).

PHYTATES

Phytic acid is found in whole grains, legumes, nuts, and seeds. Phytic acid binds to minerals such as iron, zinc and calcium, creating phytate minerals that are poorly utilized in the body. Phytic acid can be reduced by soaking grains and nuts overnight in water with the addition of an acid such as lemon juice or whey, and cooking will reduce the content too. Some sources report "serious" consequences of consuming phytic acid, yet others play down the scare mongering, saying that for there to be a serious problem, you would need to be eating a lot of untreated whole grains such as wheat germ (the phytates are in the germ component of grains) and little else.

TANNINS

Tannins are found in wine, tea, walnuts, pecans, astringent persimmons, pomegranates, vanilla, cinnamon, and cacao. Tannins are bitter and astringent— the sensation is drying to the mouth. Tannins are beneficial, with antimicrobial properties, and both phytic acid and tannins are free radical–scavenging antioxidants and have anticancer properties. Moreover, given tannins are known for reducing the absorption of iron, they are used for the condition hemochromatosis, where iron levels are abnormally high. In cases of anemia or potential anemia, it's best to avoid consuming iron-rich foods along with high-tannin foods, especially drinking black tea with an iron-containing meal.

Vitamin D

Vitamin D is important for our bones and teeth and is needed for calcium and phosphorus absorption. It is also important for balancing reproductive hormones in women and for sperm health in men. Lack of vitamin D can result in too little testosterone in men, leading to a lower sperm count, and too much testosterone in women, which can be associated with conditions such as polycystic ovarian syndrome (PCOS).

Vitamin D is best sourced from sunlight exposure on your skin, and most food sources are not smoothie friendly other than eggs—unless you want a fishy smoothie! Blergh! Vitamin D3 is what the sun helps your skin to create via the effect of UVB rays on the precursor hormone "7-dehydrocholesterol," which is then transformed into the active hormone form of vitamin D (1,25-dihydroxyvitamin D) by the kidneys and the liver. Hence, if supplementing, be sure to get vitamin D3 and not vitamin D2. Note that the precursor to vitamin D3 contains cholesterol, an essential component of all steroid hormones, which include reproductive hormones.

Reasons for vitamin D deficiency can include inadequate intake of dietary cholesterol, use of cholesterol-lowering drugs, minimal to no sunlight exposure, obesity, kidney or liver dysfunction, or intestinal disorders affecting absorption, such as Crohn's or celiac disease or gut dysbiosis (bacterial imbalance)—all of which have become more prevalent over time, as has vitamin D deficiency.

Smoothie- and fertility-friendly sources: raw eggs

Calcium

Calcium is well known for its role in healthy bones, teeth, and muscles. When it comes to fertility, calcium is more important for women than men. Calcium is an alkaline mineral, which helps form stretchy fertile cervical mucus. Sperm utilizes the calcium in these reproductive fluids to create the whip-like tail action to propel them toward the egg. Calcium in reproductive fluids also helps to trigger the cell division of an embryo.

Smoothie- and fertility-friendly sources: leafy greens, almonds, oats, calcium-enriched rice milk, sesame seeds, Brazil nuts, tahini, and chia seeds

MACRONUTRIENTS

Fats

As discussed in Chapter 2, fats are essential to fertility for both men and women. We need fats that are saturated and monounsaturated, plus omega-3 and cholesterol, for healthy cell function, to build hormones, and to absorb fat-soluble vitamins.

Smoothie- and fertility-friendly sources: young coconut flesh, avocado, macadamia, chia, flax, eggs, hemp, and walnuts. Still nutritious, but not as useful when it comes to fats, are other nuts and seeds such as cashew, almond, sesame, sunflower, and pumpkin seeds

Protein and Carbohydrates

Protein and carbohydrate requirements while preparing for conception are no different from a usual healthy diet. Protein requirements are higher for pregnant and postnatal, women and this will be discussed in more detail in subsequent chapters. It should be noted that for good blood sugar control, it's wise to eat a source of protein at each meal as this helps to slow the absorption of glucose into the bloodstream from the small intestine. This in turn makes each meal more satisfying (especially in combination with good-quality fat) so you are less likely to overeat, which is better for weight management. Being at a healthy weight aids fertility and helps to set you up for a healthy pregnancy. For similar reasons, carbohydrates in the form of starches and sugars are best kept to a minimum and are best supplied in the form of fruits, whole grains, and gluten-free grains.

Smoothie- and fertility-friendly sources of protein: raw eggs, nuts, seeds, plant-based protein powder (Miessence or Amazonia brands), leafy greens, and cooked quinoa

Smoothie- and fertility-friendly sources of carbohydrates: fruit, oats (raw or cooked as porridge), cooked quinoa, and cooked millet

PROBIOTICS

Probiotics, like fats, are essential to all aspects of preparing for, making, and raising a baby, namely due to their role in improving gut health. Probiotics are "good" or "friendly" bacteria and should make up 80 to 85 percent of all the bacteria in the gut. Even a healthy gut has some "bad" bacteria to be in the correct balance, such as candida and e-coli, which do have beneficial roles when they are present in small quantities.

When gut bacteria are out of balance, it's called "dysbiosis," with candida overgrowth being the most common problem. Most people are aware of the candida overgrowth condition called "thrush" of the vaginal/genital region, which causes discomfort, itching, and abnormal discharge. But more common is candida overgrowth in the gut, either in the small or large intestine, or both. Dysbiosis may be created due to things such as significant psychological or physical stress, exposure to radiation, drinking fluoridated and chlorinated water, poor diet (low fiber, high fat, processed foods, and sodas), excessive alcohol consumption, and use of antibiotics, contraceptive pills, and steroidal and synthetic hormonal drugs.

Dysbiosis leads to problems with digestion, liver function, and nutrient absorption; hence it can affect any number of body systems including immunity and fertility. If nutrient absorption is poor and detoxification sluggish, then this naturally has great implications on the clearance and production of hormones, and with hormone imbalance, there is greater chance of infertility in women and men.

Symptoms of dysbiosis can be wide ranging and treatment can be complex, including the elimination of sugars and yeasts, preparations to kill off bad bacteria, and probiotic supplementation to re-colonize the gut. Probiotic formulas should have many varieties of bacteria, namely different lactobacillus. My preferred brand is InLiven Probiotic Superfood, which includes all 13 strains of lactobacillus, two beneficial yeasts, and spirulina. InLiven is fermented on a base of organic legumes, grains, and vegetables for 3 weeks prior to bottling. The bacteria break down/pre-digest the food, releasing its vitamins, minerals, enzymes, and antioxidants, which are also available in the formula. Spirulina is a microalgae that is also rich in nutrients including omega-6 GLA, tyrosine, beta-carotene, calcium, and iron—all essentials for fertility—and it has all 18 amino acids in the same proportions as breast milk! The bacteria in InLiven are counted in colony-forming units (CFUs), and while the counts may not be as high as some probiotics claiming to have billions of CFUs, the bacteria in InLiven have been super-bred to withstand conditions that other preparations die quickly in, such as high heat, extreme cold, salt, food preservatives, alcohol, ascorbic acid (vitamin C), bile salts, stomach acid, and chlorine. Hence, you can take a weak probiotic that must live in the fridge, where many may die before they are put to good use, or you can take one that actively reproduces into billions in the gut. Spirulina also facilitates the reproduction of lactobacilli in the gut, which is a bonus when taking InLiven.

Smoothie- and fertility-friendly sources: Most probiotics can be conveniently added to smoothies, particularly if they come in a powder or liquid form. Many come in a capsule that you can just chuck in anyway, or you can pull it apart and empty the powder out. Given that the recommendation for optimal fertility is to remain dairy-free, probiotic-containing ingredients such as yogurt and milk kefir should also be avoided. Kefir made with water or coconut water, however, is okay.

INGREDIENTS TO AVOID

You may have noticed that the recommended ingredients so far have not contained dairy such as milk and yogurt, or soy products. Many natural fertility experts recommend being gluten-, dairy-, and soy-free for both prospective parents. Gluten should be avoided for its tendency to promote inflammation, and in untreated celiac disease, nutrient deficiencies, due to malabsorption from damage to the intestinal lining. Dairy products should be eliminated, due to their mucus-forming properties, which can include congestion of the fallopian tubes; and soy, due to its potential to disrupt reproductive and thyroid hormone function. If you are only just embarking on the journey to conceiving a baby and have no known problems with these foods, then avoiding them isn't entirely necessary. (Except soy, a food I don't recommend anyone eats; see "Liquids in Smoothies" on page 10). Smoothie recipes generally don't contain gluten anyway but frequently have a base of cow's milk, so you can easily substitute for any other milk listed in a recipe. However, if you are experiencing infertility, I do recommend you avoid dairy in your smoothies (and the rest of your diet, along with gluten and soy) because you want to stack the odds of conceiving in your favor. Remember this avoidance of certain foods need not be forever!

It is also advised to stay away from both alcohol and caffeine, which have taxing effects on the liver, and when consumed, essential fertility nutrients are depleted in order to break them down. Caffeine predominantly depletes calcium, and also iron, magnesium, vitamins A, C, and D, and B vitamins (except B12). Alcohol predominantly depletes zinc, magnesium, vitamin C, B vitamins (including B12), and also calcium, iron, and the fat-soluble vitamins A, D, and E, due to the interference alcohol has with absorption of fat. Alcohol reduces testosterone in men, affecting sperm quality and quantity. Alcohol influences the production of estrogen and progesterone in women—both essential hormones for all things reproductive, including the growth of the lining of the uterus and the ability to ovulate. Even though caffeine and alcohol are not directly relevant to the ingredients of a smoothie, the issue of nutrient depletion is. When you work hard to create healthy food and drinks, and take prenatal supplements, you don't want to shoot yourself in the foot by losing many of these nutrients to the consumption of alcohol and caffeine.

The Thyroid

The thyroid is an endocrine gland in the front of the neck that produces hormones and is very important for fertility and conception. Both an overactive and underactive thyroid can be a problem, but underactive is more common. Signs can include fatigue, feeling cold—especially in the extremities—hair loss, weight gain or difficulty losing weight, depression, constipation, irregular periods, muscular pain, poor libido, brain fog, dry skin, hoarse voice, and lower body temperature. The latter is apparent when charting your basal body temperature (first thing in the morning before moving), as it will be significantly lower than ideal, specifically below 97.7°F (36.5°C)—low temperatures interfere with the ideal conditions required for an embryo to successfully divide.

MAINTAINING A HEALTHY THYROID

Vitamins A, B12, C, D, and E, the amino acid tyrosine, and the minerals selenium, iodine, magnesium, and zinc, are all important nutrients for optimal thyroid function:

- The amino acid tyrosine and the mineral iodine are used to synthesize T3 (triiodothyronine) and T4 (thyroxine).
- Magnesium, selenium, and zinc are required to convert T4 to the active form of T3.
- Thyroid hormones are also involved in the uptake of zinc, and low zinc is linked to male and female infertility with regard to the quality of egg and sperm.
- Vitamin A regulates thyroid hormone metabolism, particularly lowering TSH (a higher TSH indicates an underactive thyroid).
- T4 contributes to the conversion of beta-carotene to vitamin A.
- Thyroid function can be negatively influenced by exposure to toxic chemicals and heavy metals—this is where vitamins C and E play an important detoxifying role as antioxidant substances.
- Vitamin D is crucial to thyroid hormone action, being required at the cellular level to facilitate their action.
- Low B12 worsens hypothyroidism and thyroid hormones that play a necessary part of B12 metabolism, so like zinc and vitamin A, inadequate B12 levels can be caught in a vicious cycle with thyroid dysfunction.
- The medium-chain fatty acids in coconut oil are great for improving metabolism and raising basal body temperature.

Iodine

The most important thyroid nutrient is iodine, and this nutrient is very important for the development of a baby's brain and nervous system. Significant iodine deficiency can cause hypothyroidism in a baby and can also cause mental retardation. Given that 50 percent of pregnancies are unplanned, this is one nutrient, like folate, that should be consumed/supplemented in adequate amounts as a childbearing woman—the RDA is 150mcg with the upper limit being 1100mcg to prevent toxicity, as more is not better. In diagnosed cases of thyroid disease, self-prescribed iodine is not advised as it can be harmful for some thyroid disorders. For more on iodine, see page 135.

Cruciferous Vegetables and Thyroid Function

Also known as brassicas, these smoothie- and salad-friendly cruciferous green leafy vegetables include kale, bok choy, cabbage, and radish tops. Other brassicas include broccoli, Brussels sprouts, and cauliflower. These vegetables can be a problem for an underactive thyroid because they interfere with the uptake of iodine, an essential nutrient for thyroid function. These vegetables are also important for liver detoxification, which includes getting rid of excess estrogen. Thankfully, while the goitrogenic effect of brassicas is significant when they are eaten raw, their detoxifying effect is still available when cooked, so there is no need to cease eating them completely if there is an issue with a preexisting underactive thyroid. With normal thyroid function, there is no need to be overly concerned about avoiding brassicas at all, except raw brassicas daily is not ideal for reasons of potential interference with iodine.

THE THYROID AND FERTILITY

A healthy thyroid is absolutely essential for a woman's fertility, and it's also important for men. Underactive thyroid conditions are less common in men, but will have the effect of altering the function of the reproductive organs via hormone imbalance, not unlike what happens in women. The result is poor sperm morphology and motility, and reduced semen volume. All of which are a problem when half of a healthy conception is a set of strong and healthy swimmers. In women, T3 and T4 support FSH (follicle stimulating hormone) and LH (luteinizing hormone) to stimulate the ovary for egg release, and T3 stimulates luteal cells to release progesterone. Moreover, vitamins A and B12 plus zinc are essential for fertility, and the thyroid is involved in absorption of these nutrients.

If you are experiencing unexplained infertility, it is worth having your thyroid function checked, which involves looking at TSH (thyroid stimulating hormone), T3, T4, and thyroid antibodies. My mildly raised antibodies and elevated TSH were successfully treated with natural medicine. Some people, however, require thyroid hormone replacement and this includes those trying to conceive. These decisions will be made between you and your treating health practitioner.

In my case, 3 years of infertility was unexplained by the medical profession. It was my naturopath that diagnosed an underactive thyroid, only mildly, but enough to negatively influence my cycle. I was already living a healthy lifestyle that included being gluten- and dairy-free (due to intolerance), I consumed very little soy, ate organically, had eliminated chemicals from personal care, cosmetics, and cleaning products from my home, and minimized EMR (electromagnetic radiation) exposure. With herbal medicine and specific nutrients to boost my thyroid function, and strictly avoiding foods that tend to make it worse, I corrected my hormone imbalance over 6 months. Where I was going wrong with food was the use of raw cruciferous veg in my green smoothies.

Estrogen and Progesterone

Estrogen is a group of hormones that are present in women more than men. In women they are responsible for feminizing the female body and stimulating the growth of the lining of the uterus during a menstrual cycle. In men it aids maturation of sperm.

In women, progesterone helps maintain the growth of the uterine lining (endometrium) and prepares it for egg implantation. Progesterone levels remain high and rise during pregnancy to keep the endometrium thick, and this nourishes the placenta. Progesterone also prevents lactation because it opposes prolactin, the hormone necessary for milk production. A lack of progesterone is a common problem with infertility, affecting the length of the menstrual cycle, with short and irregular-length cycles common. A lack of progesterone often goes hand in hand with thyroid dysfunction and can also affect mood, weight, and libido.

Progesterone is usually assessed via blood test on day 21 of the menstrual cycle, because that is when the peak amount of progesterone is produced—assuming you have a 28-day cycle and you are ovulating. If you don't, a day-21 test won't be accurate. Progesterone will peak 7 days after you ovulate, so knowing when and if you ovulate is necessary to accurately test progesterone. Ovulation test kits are available, or you can take your temperature every morning and take note of cervical mucus changes over your cycle. Temperature rises and stays elevated after ovulation due to a rise in progesterone, so this method tells that you have already ovulated. Change in mucus from a sticky paste to a stretchy egg white–like substance, occurs as ovulation approaches.

In men, mood, energy, libido, muscle mass, erections, and sperm count are all influenced by progesterone. Progesterone is the precursor hormone to testosterone, the key male reproductive hormone that masculinizes men and plays a significant role in sperm production. Progesterone is also the precursor hormone to estrogen, so if progesterone isn't functioning correctly, it affects the whole system.

ESTROGEN DOMINANCE

Estrogen dominance is something that can affect both men and women. It means estrogen levels are higher than ideal with simultaneous lower levels of progesterone. The issue with excess estrogen is significant when it comes to fertility and trying to conceive.

Estrogen dominance is thought to occur because there are additional sources of estrogen other than that produced for reproductive purposes. First, aromatase enzyme converts testosterone to estrogen in a process called aromatization, and this enzyme is present in many tissues, particularly fat, so if overweight or obese, aromatization is likely to occur. Natural aromatase inhibitors include olive oil, chamomile, and the antioxidant quercetin.

Second, there is the presence of xenoestrogens, which are substances that mimic real estrogens. They come from the environment: plastics, pollution, chemicals in cosmetics, and personal care and cleaning products. Hence, this is why it's so important for our well-being and especially fertility to detoxify the home, as well as what we put on our bodies, not just what we put in our bodies. Xenoestrogens lack a "methyl" group to their structure, so anything that can donate a methyl group helps to eliminate them from the body. This process is called methylation. Foods that contain betaine and choline are helpful for this purpose (as are methylated forms of B vitamins, as discussed earlier). To eliminate excess estrogen we need a healthy liver, so a diet rich in antioxidants plant foods is essential. Moreover, cessation of chemically laden processed foods, alcohol, and caffeine are essential to optimal liver function.

Third, if under stress and producing excessive amounts of cortisol from the adrenal glands, this will negatively influence hormone balance, particularly the production of progesterone.

Conditions in women such as endometriosis and polycystic ovary syndrome (PCOS) involve an element of estrogen dominance and will hence benefit from diet and lifestyle changes that reduce xenoestrogen exposure and elimination of excess estrogens (plus other strategies to boost progesterone). The hormonal malfunctioning with these conditions is quite complex, particularly with PCOS, in which lack of ovulation is another reason for high estrogen and low progesterone. Further discussion of these conditions is beyond the scope of this book; however, if you have either of these conditions, I highly recommend finding a practitioner experienced in treating them naturally, as it's possible to do so.

Smoothie- and fertility-friendly ingredients that oppose estrogen dominance: apples, berries, cherries, citrus, grapes, and parsley for quercetin. Egg yolk, chard, collards, peanuts, and sunflower seeds for choline. Beets and goji berries for betaine. Leafy greens, berries, turmeric, ginger, lemons, limes, beets, and brassicas for liver health. (However, avoid raw brassicas if you have an underactive thyroid, as discussed in "Cruciferous Vegetables and Thyroid Function" on page 69.)

OPTIMIZING TESTOSTERONE AND PROGESTERONE

Vitamins A, B6, C, D, E, the minerals zinc and magnesium, cholesterol, protein, and healthy fats are all very important for fertility, including for progesterone and testosterone production and function. We need cholesterol to make testosterone, progesterone, and vitamin D, so low cholesterol, particularly due to using statin drugs, and/or minimal skin exposure to sunlight may contribute to problems with fertility. Protein is available to some degree in all whole foods, but not many plant foods are "complete proteins," which means they don't have all eight essential amino acids. All of these nutrients have been discussed so far, except vitamin B6, an important nutrient for a myriad of bodily functions including mental health, energy, and hormone balance.

Smoothie- and fertility-friendly sources: avocado, bananas, carrots, leafy greens (especially spinach, kale, and collards), fennel, prunes, dried apricots, sweet potato, beets, sunflower seeds, and eggs

Genetics, Chemistry, and Fertility

There are many, many factors that can influence fertility. Many aren't common, such as rare genetic mutations that can affect hormone balance or blood clotting. Others are more common than you may realize, such as thyroid disorders. If you have been struggling with becoming pregnant, the following topics may be of interest to you and are worth getting tested for.

MTHFR MUTATION

MTHFR (or methylenetetrahydrofolate reductase) is a gene discovered as part of the human genome project that was completed in 2003. Forty to fifty different mutations have been reported, but the two problematic mutations are called C677T and A1298C, which are passed from parents to children. Their presence means that the enzyme (also called MTHFR) that converts folic acid to its usable form, methylfolate, is less efficient. It also negatively impacts the conversion or "methylation" of vitamins B2 and B6 to their methyl forms (riboflavin-5-phosphate and pyroxidal-5-phosphate, respectively), as well as B12.

The mutation C677T is associated with cardiovascular problems, including high homocysteine and clotting disorders, and A1298C is associated more with neurological and mental health problems. Both can be associated with infertility and miscarriages.

METHYLATION

Methylation is the term to describe the transfer of a "methyl" molecule from one substance to another. In the case of vitamin B12, a methyl group from trimethylglycine (TMG) can "methylate" cyanocobalamin to methylcobalamin (not in one step but overall). Methylation involving folate and B12 is essential for DNA synthesis, for detoxification, and for fat and cholesterol metabolism, so a deficiency of either can have huge repercussions for health generally and for fertility, conception, and pregnancy, given their subsequent roles in hormone production and regulation, and healthy cell division. Vitamin B2 and B6 also require methylation. As discussed earlier, vitamin B6 is needed for a multitude of bodily functions, especially hormone balance, as it helps the liver process excess estrogen and helps boost progesterone. B2 is important for energy production alongside the other B vitamins, as well as being great for the liver and for iron metabolism. So even in the absence of the MTHFR mutation, diets with plentiful methyl groups are very important! TMG, otherwise known as betaine, can methylate three things as it has three methyl groups, which is rather handy! Choline is a precursor to TMG and is part of the B vitamin group—though not strictly a vitamin, it is an essential component of phospholipids that make up all of the human body's cell membranes. Choline is required for a healthy liver via assistance with fat metabolism, a healthy nervous system, and also for the prevention of neural tube defects via its role as a methyl group donor.

Smoothie- and fertility-friendly sources of choline: raw egg yolks, sunflower seeds, and peanuts

Smoothie- and fertility-friendly sources of vitamin B2: almonds, spinach, sweet potato, pumpkin, beet greens, mint, spirulina, maple syrup, raw eggs

Note: If you have problems methylating due to having MTHFR, then you will need to take specific methylated B vitamin supplements to address deficiencies.

HOMOCYSTEINE

Homocysteine is a substance that is part of a series of cellular reactions in the body that starts with consuming the amino acid methionine in the diet and converting it to SAMe (s-adenosylmethionine) and glutathione. The former is particularly important for mental health, and the latter essential for liver detoxification. If these reactions get stuck because nutrients or enzymes are missing or lacking, then homocysteine levels rise, and high levels are associated with many conditions and illnesses, including infertility, and pregnancy complications such as preeclampsia, miscarriages, birth defects, low birth weight babies, premature babies, and poor placental function. Nutrients that lower homocysteine include methylated forms of B2, B6, B9 (folate), and B12, magnesium, zinc, and TMG—plenty of methyl donors are required because homocysteine lacks a methyl group. Beets are a great smoothie-friendly source of betaine (TMG). Beets also contain betalain pigments that help with glutathione function, so beets, including root, stems, and leaves, are excellent for the liver, and a healthy liver is a must for hormone balance and fertility!

Other smoothie- and fertility-friendly, glutathione-boosting foods: chia, flax, avocado, peaches, cinnamon, cardamom, watermelon, walnuts, Brazil nuts, sunflower seeds, cabbage, and kale

For years, despite consuming B12 in my diet and supplementing with cyanocobalamin, my B12 was always on the low side and even dropped below normal—which according to my pathology lab was below 180pmol/L. In parts of the world such as Europe and Japan, normal is over 500 according to their pathology labs. I was very low at 165 at one stage and subsequently struggled to get anywhere near 500. Mind you, I was asymptomatic in terms of neurological signs and energy levels, but I was infertile. I remember a very rude doctor seeing this result who verbally attacked me, assuming I was being an irresponsible vegan—which I wasn't! I was vegetarian at the time, but did eat small amounts of dairy, ate plenty of eggs, took lots of probiotics, and was taking B12 supplements. It wasn't until years later that my naturopath wanted this tested alongside MTHFR and homocysteine as part of a very thorough screening of my health to figure out why I couldn't conceive. Unsurprisingly, it came back with a single C667T defect and my homocysteine was 9.1, which was still within normal ranges but too high for fertility. I was subsequently started on methylated B vitamins such as those described already, and I ceased any that were in a form I couldn't metabolize well. My B12 then rose over 500 and has kept rising, and my homocysteine lowered to 6.6—I believe this played a big part in restoring my fertility hand in hand with improving my thyroid function.

Dealing with Nutrient Thieves

The importance of nutrition is clear when it comes to fertility. It's also important to know how nutrients may be unnecessarily robbed from your body and when during your monthly cycle you require greater nourishment.

THE PILL

Women coming off the contraceptive pill with the intention of getting pregnant should know that the pill results in losses of important nutrients for fertility including B vitamins (particularly important are folic acid, B6, and B12), vitamins C and E, magnesium, and zinc—all important nutrients for making hormones as discussed in this chapter. Some women are advised 3 months is sufficient to wait after coming off the pill before trying to conceive, but remember it takes 4 months for an egg to mature—ideally in a nutrient-rich environment—so coming off the pill earlier than this is paramount, and it should be at least 6 months, if not longer.

THE 2-WEEK WAIT

If you are actively trying to conceive, you will experience each month, the trepidation of the "2-week wait" after mid-cycle sexy time. Either your period arrives or it doesn't. As discussed previously, due to the rise of hormones in the second half of the cycle, the liver works harder and more nutrients are required. So this time of the month is a time to be extra kind to yourself through avoiding excessive exertion and stress, and encouraging relaxation and extra sleep. Furthermore, provide extra nutrients via careful attention to your diet—and smoothies!—supplying foods that are magnesium rich, blood building and warming to your uterus, and cleansing to the liver. Iron in combination with vitamins B6, B12, and folic acid are "blood building," meaning they are essential components of red blood cell formation.

Smoothie- and fertility-friendly blood-building and liver-cleansing foods: leafy greens, beets, carrots, apricots, avocado, dates, prunes, citrus, figs, nuts and seeds, raw eggs (especially the yolks), bananas, lemons, limes, cruciferous vegetables, cardamom, alfalfa, ginger, licorice, quinoa, and oats; plus warming spices such as ginger and cinnamon

The Smoothies

As part of my research for this book I created a detailed survey that was completed by hundreds of mothers. According to this survey, smoothies being made for two adults only made up 15 percent of respondents, and partners were more likely to have a smoothie as a snack, versus women mostly having them as a meal. Hence, the following recipes make approximately 500ml/2 cups as a large serving for one. If sharing smoothies with your partner, simply double the recipe. Nutritionally, you both need similar nutrients for different reproductive functions anyway, so they will benefit men as well as women.

Please note that recipes will vary in thickness and sweetness according to the choice of ingredients, and this will vary further, particularly with flavor, due to differences between seasons and produce quality. Should a recipe turn out thicker than you would like, add some more liquid; if it's not sweet enough, add some sweetener; if you would like a cold smoothie, use some ice in place of the liquid component. If you haven't read the introductory chapters before attempting my recipes, please go back and read them, particularly Chapter 1, "The Art and Science of Smoothies," which has detailed guidelines for my smoothie creations. All of the recipes for preconception care are free of dairy, gluten, and soy.

All recipes in this chapter yield 2 cups (500ml) and serve 1.

THYROID-FRIENDLY SMOOTHIES

The following smoothies are well suited for optimizing thyroid health, which as we know is essential for fertility. Moreover, they are particularly good for those with underactive thyroid function, featuring ingredients rich in vitamins A, C, E, and B12, tyrosine, selenium, iodine, magnesium, and zinc.

Goitrogenic ingredients are not included in these recipes, which most importantly exclude soy and raw brassicas. Greens can be steamed to eliminate the majority of the goitrogens, but there is still enough variety to use other greens in raw form, which makes them taste better in smoothies anyway. To a lesser extent, the following smoothie-friendly foods are mild goitrogens and won't be included either: peanuts, flax, strawberries, pears, peaches, spinach, sweet potato, and millet.

Coconut and Papaya Pudding

1 cup papaya

juice of 1 lime

¼ cup coconut flesh and ¾ cup coconut water from a drinking coconut

Melon and Berry Bonanza

1 cup cantaloupe

1½ cups raspberries

1 tablespoon chia seeds

Pineapple Pizzazz

1 cup pineapple, fresh or frozen small pieces

1 kiwi including peel, halved

1 medium Persian cucumber, quartered

handful of mint leaves

Sweet Potato Sensation

½ cup steamed or pureed sweet potato or pumpkin

1 banana, fresh or frozen and sliced

1 tablespoon tahini

¼ teaspoon ground Sri Lankan cinnamon

pinch of ground nutmeg

2 medjool dates, pitted

1 cup non-dairy milk

1 egg (optional)

Citrus Celebration

2 packed cups orange or mandarin orange segments

zest and flesh from ½ lemon (or all of the lemon if the pith is thin)

2 tablespoons hemp seeds

sweeten to taste

handful of parsley (optional)

Figgy-Grape Goodness

½ packed cup fresh figs

1 packed cup seedless grapes

¾ cup almond milk

10 raw cashews

¼ teaspoon ground Sri Lankan cinnamon

¼ inch slice fresh ginger

3 ice cubes

Popping with Pink

½ cup pomegranate juice*

¼ cup diced raw beet

½ cup coconut flesh and ¾ cup coconut water from a drinking coconut

handful of parsley (optional)

*To juice pomegranates, blend the seeds for 10–15 seconds then strain through a fine sieve.

Muesli in a Glass

½ cup raw, wheat-free muesli*

1 banana

1 cup non-dairy milk

1 egg (optional)

*If time permits, soak the muesli in the milk overnight in the fridge, which will result in a creamier smoothie made the next day.

Beta-Carotene Blitz

1 banana, frozen and sliced

½ cup fresh or steamed apricots

1 cup carrot juice

1 heaping tablespoon sunflower seeds*

1 teaspoon vanilla extract or paste, or ½ vanilla bean, or thin slice of ginger

1 egg (optional)

*Ideally, soak seeds overnight in water, then drain and rinse before use.

Mango Passion

1 banana

1 cup mango flesh (about 1 mango)

¾ cup non-dairy milk or water

2 tablespoons hemp seeds or 5 macadamias

pulp of 1 passion fruit*

*Blend all except passion fruit, which you stir through at the end by hand.

Spice Girls

2 tablespoons raw oats plus ½ cup water or milk, or ½ cup cooked oats, quinoa, or millet

1 banana, fresh or frozen and sliced

¼ teaspoon ground Sri Lankan cinnamon

pinch of ground nutmeg

pinch of ground cardamom

1 teaspoon vanilla extract or paste, or ½ vanilla bean

1 tablespoon maple syrup

1 cup almond milk

1 egg (optional)

METHYLATION SMOOTHIES

The following smoothie recipes are designed to facilitate methylation pathways and include nutrients such as B2, B6, folate (B9), B12, magnesium, zinc, and choline. If you have been diagnosed with high homocysteine levels, estrogen dominance, or B12 deficiency, or have a history of miscarriage or pregnancy complications such as birth defects, preeclampsia, or premature labor, then these smoothies are for you.

Betalain Bonus

½ cup diced raw beet

1 cup pitted cherries

¾ cup coconut water

1 tablespoon chia seeds

1 bulb baby bok choy, trimmed and well washed

Nuts for Pumpkin

½ cup steamed or pureed sweet potato or pumpkin

1 banana, frozen and sliced

8 raw pecan or walnut halves*

1 cup non-dairy milk

maple syrup to taste

1 egg (optional)

*Ideally, soak nuts overnight in water, then drain and rinse before use. This will not only aid digestibility but also reduce bitterness of walnuts or pecans.

Citrus and Melon Mover

1 packed cup orange or mandarin orange segments

1 cup cantaloupe or honeydew melon

1–2 handfuls of spinach

Strawberry Fields Forever

2 frozen bananas, sliced

1½ cups/1 punnet strawberries with hulls

2 tablespoons hemp seeds

2 sprigs mint leaves

Better Than a Snickers Bar

2 frozen bananas, sliced

¾ cup non-dairy milk or water

1 tablespoon natural peanut butter

1 tablespoon raw cacao and tiny pinch salt

1 egg (optional)

Mango Vanilla Va-Voom

1 cup mango flesh (about 1 mango)

¼ cup coconut flesh and ¾ cup coconut water from a drinking coconut

1 teaspoon vanilla extract or paste, or ½ vanilla bean

handful of Swiss chard (optional)

1 egg (optional)

Goji Greatness

2 tablespoons raw oats plus 3 tablespoons goji berries soaked in 1½ cups non-dairy milk overnight in the fridge

1 banana, fresh or frozen and sliced

2 tablespoons coconut cream

1 teaspoon vanilla extract or paste, or ½ vanilla bean

1 egg (optional)

Fantastic Fennel

2 bananas

2 handfuls of fennel tops

zest from ¼ lemon*

8 ice cubes

honey or stevia to taste

*Use a vegetable peeler to remove zest.

Figgy Fever

1 packed cup fresh figs

¾ cup almond milk

¼ teaspoon ground Sri Lankan cinnamon

4 ice cubes

1 tablespoon chia seeds

Papaya Perfection

1 banana

1 cup papaya

squeeze of lemon or lime juice

4 ice cubes

OPTIMIZING HORMONE SMOOTHIES

The following smoothie recipes are all about optimizing the key hormones for fertility for women and men—progesterone and testosterone——which require vitamins A, C, E, D, magnesium, zinc, good fats, and protein.

Pine-Lime-Kiwi Kooler

1 cup pineapple, fresh or frozen small pieces

1 kiwi with skin, halved

juice or flesh of ½ lime

¾ cup coconut water

Enzyme Frenzy

1 cup papaya

1 cup freshly squeezed orange juice

¼ avocado

Protein-Rich Peach Melba

¾ cup fresh* or steamed peach halves

½ cup fresh or frozen raspberries

1 teaspoon vanilla extract or paste, or ½ vanilla bean

1 cup non-dairy milk

1 heaping tablespoon pumpkin and/or sunflower seeds**

1 egg (optional)

*It's essential that fresh peaches are ripe, sweet, and juicy.

**Ideally, soak seeds overnight, discard water, and rinse well.

Crazy for Carrots

1 frozen banana, sliced, or ½ mango

½ cup raw or steamed carrot

1 heaping tablespoon pumpkin and/or sunflower seeds*

¼ inch slice fresh ginger

1 cup non-dairy milk

1 egg (optional)

*Ideally, soak seeds overnight, discard water, and rinse well.

Chocolate Bircher Porridge

2 tablespoons raw rolled oats

1¼ cups non-dairy milk (not coconut)

2 dried figs

2 pitted prunes

2 dried apricots

1 tablespoon raw cacao

tiny pinch of salt

2 tablespoons hemp seeds

Combine all ingredients in a bowl in the fridge overnight, and then blend the contents the next day.

Magnificent Mango

1 cup mango flesh (about 1 mango)

1 cup non-dairy milk

1 serving plant-based protein powder

1 teaspoon vanilla extract or paste, or ½ vanilla bean

Wow for Watermelon

1½ cups watermelon

1½ cups frozen blueberries

1 tablespoon chia seeds

Packed with Protein

2 bananas, fresh or frozen and sliced

1 tablespoon hulled tahini

1 serving plant-based protein powder

1 tablespoon raw cacao

tiny pinch of salt

1 cup non-dairy milk or coconut water

1 egg (optional)

Plums-a-Plenty

¾ cup plum halves (preferably satsuma)*

¾ cup nectarines halves*

thin slice of fresh ginger

4 raw walnut or pecan halves**

¾ cup non-dairy milk

maple syrup to taste

*It's essential that stone fruit is ripe, sweet, and juicy.

**Ideally, soak overnight, drain, and rinse before blending—this will aid digestion, as well as improve the flavor of the nuts once blended.

Citrus Sizzler

1 packed cup orange segments

zest and flesh from ½ lemon (or all of the lemon if the pith is thin)

¼ cup coconut flesh and ¾ cup coconut water from a drinking coconut

handful of parsley (optional)

Apricot and Peach Passion

½ cup fresh apricots*

½ cup fresh peaches*

1 cup almond milk

¼ avocado

pinch of ground cardamom

1 teaspoon vanilla extract or paste, or ½ vanilla bean

sweeten to taste

1 egg (optional)

*It's essential that stone fruit is ripe, sweet, and juicy.

Pomegranate Popper

juice of 1 pomegranate (about ½ cup)* and retain 2 tablespoons seeds**

1 cup pitted cherries, fresh or frozen

2 tablespoons hemp seeds

1 tablespoon chia seeds

¾ cup coconut water

*To make pomegranate juice, blend seeds for 10–15 seconds, and then strain through a fine sieve.

**Stir the tablespoon of pomegranate seeds through the smoothie by hand after blending—make sure you "chew" this smoothie.

Full of Passion

1 banana, fresh or frozen and sliced

1 cup fresh pineapple pieces

1 heaping tablespoon sunflower seeds**

¾ cup coconut water

pulp of 1 passion fruit*

*Blend all except passion fruit, which you stir through at the end by hand.

**Ideally, soak seeds overnight, discard water, and rinse well.

Strawberry Shortcake

2 tablespoons raw oats plus ½ cup of water or milk, or ½ cup of cooked oats, quinoa, or millet

1½ cups/1 punnet strawberries with hulls

¼ inch slice raw beet

zest from ¼ lemon*

½ cup coconut milk

3 medjool dates, pitted

*Use a vegetable peeler to remove zest.

Peanuts for Pumpkin

½ cup steamed or pureed sweet potato or pumpkin

1 banana, fresh or frozen and sliced

1 tablespoon natural peanut butter

1 cup non-dairy milk

½ teaspoon ground Sri Lankan cinnamon

½ teaspoon ground turmeric (optional)

1 egg (optional)

LIVER-CLEANSING SMOOTHIES

A healthy liver is essential for hormone balance and detoxification. Both hormone imbalance and dealing with a toxic load (e.g., pesticide exposure from non-organic foods, synthetic chemical-based cosmetics, alcohol, caffeine, the pill) can contribute to infertility or pregnancy complications. The following smoothie recipes are all about keeping that liver in tip-top shape and include antioxidant nutrients, such as glutathione, glucosinolates, chlorophyll, and carotenoids, as well as foods that boost glutathione function.

Spicy Brazilian

1 cup pineapple, fresh or small frozen pieces

4 Brazil nuts*

1 tablespoon hemps seeds

1 cup almond milk

pinch of cardamom

½ teaspoon ground turmeric

1 egg yolk (optional)

*Ideally, soak nuts overnight, discard water, and rinse well.

Just Peachy

¾ cup fresh peach halves*

1 banana, fresh or frozen and sliced

zest from ¼ lemon**

¾ cup non-dairy milk

1 bulb baby bok choy (optional), trimmed and well washed

*It's essential that peaches are ripe, sweet, and juicy.

**Use a vegetable peeler to remove zest.

Choc-Cherry Chillax

1 banana, fresh or frozen and sliced

½ cup pitted cherries

¼ avocado

1 medjool date, pitted

¾ cup non-dairy milk

1 egg (optional)

Papaya Lime Luxury

1 cup papaya

juice or flesh of ½ lime

1 cup coconut water

3 tablespoons coconut cream

handful of spinach (optional)

Lemon Love

zest and flesh from 1 medium lemon (or all of the lemon if the pith is thin)*

2 bananas, frozen and sliced

1 heaping tablespoon sunflower seeds**

¾ cup coconut water

handful of parsley (optional)

sweeten to taste

*Use a vegetable peeler to remove zest.

**Ideally, soak seeds overnight in water, then drain and rinse before use.

Melon and Beet Brilliance

2 cups watermelon

¼ cup chopped beet

1 tablespoon chia seeds

handful of beet greens (optional)

Orange Zinger

2 bananas or 2 pears, or 1 of each

¾ cup carrot juice

¼ inch fresh ginger

4 Brazil nuts*

½ teaspoon ground turmeric (optional)

1 egg yolk (optional)

*Ideally, soak nuts overnight, discard water, and rinse well.

Clever Carrots

½ cup diced raw or steamed carrot*

1 banana, fresh or frozen and sliced

10 raw cashews

½ teaspoon ground turmeric

½ teaspoon ground Sri Lankan cinnamon

1 teaspoon vanilla extract or paste, or ½ vanilla bean

1 cup non-dairy milk

1–2 Chinese cabbage leaves (optional)

1 egg yolk (optional)

*Raw carrot will take longer to blend.

Vanilla Dream

2 bananas, frozen and sliced

¾ cup coconut milk

2 teaspoons vanilla extract or paste, or 1 vanilla bean, halved

1 egg yolk (optional)

Princess Peach

1 cup fresh* or steamed peaches

6 raw macadamias

1 teaspoon vanilla extract or paste, or ½ vanilla bean

¼ inch slice fresh ginger

1 cup non-dairy milk

sweeten to taste

1 egg yolk (optional)

*It's essential that peaches are ripe, sweet, and juicy.

Detox Diva

1 cup beet and celery juice

1 Granny Smith apple, cut into 8 pieces

6 raw walnut halves*

handful of parsley (optional)

3 ice cubes

*Ideally, soak overnight, drain, and rinse before blending—this will aid digestion as well as improve the flavor of the walnuts once blended.

Love Your Liver

zest and flesh from ½ lemon*

1 cup orange segments

¼ avocado

¾ cup coconut water

3 ice cubes

sweeten to taste

handful of kale (optional)

*Use a vegetable peeler to remove zest.

Sweet Sensation

1½ cups watermelon

1½ cups/1 punnet strawberries with hulls

handful of Swiss chard (optional)

LUTEAL PHASE SMOOTHIES

Nutrient requirements in the second half of your menstrual cycle, also known as the luteal phase, are much higher due to rising hormone levels and result in a harder workload by the liver. Hence, smoothies in the luteal phase require liver-boosting and blood-building nutrients such as plant-based antioxidants, iron, B6, B12, and folate, as well as plenty of magnesium and zinc.

B Vitamin Booster

2 bananas, fresh or frozen and sliced

zest and flesh from ½ lemon*

6 raw macadamias

¾ cup coconut water

1–2 handfuls of spinach (optional)

1 egg yolk (optional)

*Use a vegetable peeler to remove zest.

Fabulous Fennel

2 bananas, fresh or frozen and sliced

tops of ½ fennel bulb or 1 teaspoon ground fennel seeds*

zest from ¼ lemon**

¾ cup coconut milk or coconut water

*Grind with a spice grinder or mortar and pestle.

**Use a vegetable peeler to remove zest.

Lemon Slice

½ cup coconut flesh and ¾ cup coconut water from a drinking coconut

zest and flesh from ½ lemon*

1 tablespoon chia seeds

3 medjool dates, pitted

3 ice cubes

1–2 leaves Chinese cabbage or 1 bulb baby bok choy (optional), trimmed and well washed

*Use a vegetable peeler to remove zest.

Fig-tastic

1 cup fresh figs, stem tip removed

¾ cup frozen seedless grapes

¾ cup almond milk

6 raw walnut or pecan halves*

handful of romaine lettuce (optional)

*Ideally, soak overnight, drain, and rinse before blending—this will aid digestion as well as improve the flavor of the nuts once blended.

Pear and Carrot Cleanser

½ cup steamed carrot

1 pear, quartered (must be soft and juicy)

½ teaspoon ground turmeric

¼ inch slice fresh ginger

2 tablespoons hemp seeds

2 medjool dates, pitted

1 cup coconut water

handful of alfalfa sprouts (optional)

Peanut Butter and Banana Bonanza

2 bananas, fresh or frozen and sliced

1 tablespoon natural peanut butter

¾ cup non-dairy milk or water

handful of butter lettuce

1 egg yolk (optional)

½ teaspoon ground turmeric (optional)

Apricot and Cardamom Classic

1 frozen banana, sliced

½ cup fresh* or steamed apricot halves

1 tablespoon almond butter

¼ teaspoon ground cardamom

1 cup non-dairy milk or water

handful of Swiss chard (optional)

1 egg yolk (optional)

*It's essential that fresh apricots are ripe, sweet, and juicy.

Chocolate Pudding

2 tablespoons raw rolled oats plus ½ cup water or milk, or ½ cup cooked oats, quinoa, or millet

1 banana, fresh or frozen and sliced

¼ avocado

1 tablespoon of raw cacao

tiny pinch of salt

3 medjool dates, pitted

1 cup non-dairy milk

1 egg yolk (optional)

handful of spinach (optional)

Papaya and Mango Madness

¾ cup papaya

¾ cup mango flesh

¾ cup coconut water

squeeze of lemon juice

Magnificent Melon with Ginger and Lime

2½ cups watermelon

flesh or juice of ½ lime

¼ inch slice fresh ginger

1 tablespoon chia seeds

handful of kale (optional)

Antioxidant Overload

¼ cup diced raw or steamed beet

1 cup frozen blueberries

¾ cup almond milk

10 raw cashews

1 tablespoon chia seeds

handful of beet leaves (optional)

Peaches and Cream

1 banana, fresh or frozen and sliced

¾ cup fresh* or steamed peaches

4 Brazil nuts**

1 tablespoon hemp seeds

1 teaspoon vanilla extract or paste, or ½ vanilla bean

1 cup non-dairy milk or water

1 egg yolk (optional)

*It's essential that fresh peaches are ripe, sweet, and juicy.

**Ideally, soak nuts overnight, discard water, and rinse well.

Choc-Mint Magic

2 bananas, frozen and sliced

¼ avocado

1 tablespoon raw cacao plus tiny pinch of salt

3–4 sprigs mint leaves

¾ cup non-dairy milk

1 medjool date, pitted

1 egg yolk (optional)

Muesli Smoothie

½ cup raw wheat-free muesli

1 cup non-dairy milk

1 banana

1 egg yolk (optional)

*If time permits, soak the muesli in the milk overnight in the fridge.

Silly for Citrus

½ cup steamed or raw carrot

1 cup orange segments

1 tablespoon tahini

2 medjool dates, pitted

¾ cup non-dairy milk or water

¼ teaspoon ground Sri Lankan cinnamon

1 teaspoon vanilla extract or paste, or ½ vanilla bean

handful of parsley (optional)

Smashing Spices

2 bananas, fresh or frozen and sliced

3 tablespoons coconut cream

1 teaspoon vanilla extract or paste, or ½ vanilla bean

¼ teaspoon ground turmeric

¼ teaspoon ground Sri Lankan cinnamon

pinch of ground cardamom

pinch of ground cloves

pinch of ground nutmeg

¾ cup non-dairy milk

1 egg yolk (optional)

Digestive Devotion

2 cups beet and carrot juice

¼ inch slice fresh ginger

handful of beet greens

This smoothie will have more of a juice consistency but has fiber from the greens.

CHAPTER 4

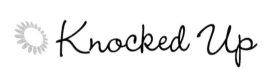 *Knocked Up*

Congratulations! You're pregnant! Such exciting times!

If you're in the 50 percent of women who have an unplanned pregnancy, even if you're a few months along, it's never too late to make healthy choices for you and your growing baby. For those where a pregnancy was planned, assuming you made choices such as consuming extra folate and iodine, and ceasing alcohol while preparing for and trying to conceive, these behaviors should continue. In fact, all of the nutrients relevant for preconception are still relevant for pregnancy, though some are more, or less, important and their roles may be somewhat different. Nutrition of the mother is actually more important during preconception than during pregnancy. For instance, in times of war when there is lack of quality food, it has been observed that babies born to mothers who were pregnant during these times had healthier babies than women who became pregnant during these times, which emphasizes the importance of egg and sperm quality. Of course, if you have the choice, be as healthy as possible during preconception *and* pregnancy.

If you've started reading this book while pregnant, and have jumped to this chapter, please read Chapter 3, "Making Babies," as there is information there that is relevant to this and the following chapters that isn't repeated in as much detail. Also, given the emphasis on the importance of preconception care, if this is something you haven't done, don't worry or stress about what you perhaps should have done differently. Any change that benefits the health of you and your baby is fantastic, and *right now* is the best time to do this!

Pregnancy Do's and Don'ts

In terms of do's and don'ts during pregnancy, the lists can be expansive. The most important don'ts are eating foods like raw eggs, soft cheeses, raw seafood, and commercially prepared salads, for risk of introducing pathogens that may give you food poisoning. Your immune system is not as strong while pregnant in order to prevent your body from rejecting the growing embryo. Food poisoning can result in miscarriage early on and can affect the baby's ability to thrive and gain weight during the pregnancy. The only relevant ingredients to avoid for smoothies are raw eggs, and avoid green smoothies if you haven't prepared them yourself.

During preconception it is advised to cease dairy and gluten, particularly if you have had trouble conceiving. If you have a known intolerance or allergy, you won't consume them whether you are pregnant or not, but there is no need to keep avoiding these things once pregnant if you are usually fine with them. Therefore, the use of cow's milk in smoothies is perfectly fine if that is your preference when "any milk" is listed in a recipe. The more diverse your diet is during pregnancy the better. Food and drink you consume will flavor the amniotic fluid surrounding your baby, and the baby has taste buds, so they will be exposed to various tastes in utero, which are believed to benefit your child's palate when they are established on solids and are eating family foods. Moreover, it is not necessary to avoid anything out of fear of your baby developing an allergy. The evidence currently doesn't support that eating allergenic foods like dairy or peanuts will give your child a dairy or peanut allergy.

Avoiding alcohol and caffeine is recommended for the same reasons as during preconception—namely, because both deplete essential nutrients like zinc, magnesium, calcium, iron, B vitamins, and vitamins A, C, D, and E. They also tax the liver in order to break them down—and remember, we need a healthy liver for balanced hormones; hormone production is significant during pregnancy! Alcohol crosses the placenta and will enter a baby's bloodstream. Excessive drinking has been clearly linked to fetal alcohol syndrome, including stunted growth and organ damage, particularly if drinking in the first trimester of pregnancy when a baby's liver is far less mature than later in the pregnancy and much less capable of processing it. All major health organizations around the world, including the American Academy of Pediatrics (AAP) in the United States, National Health and Medical Research Council (NHMRC) in Australia, and Department of Health (DOH) in the UK, state there is no proven safe level of alcohol consumption for pregnant women and women trying to get pregnant, and recommend that *no alcohol be consumed*. Despite this, I was advised by my obstetrician that the odd glass here and there was fine, and a friend of mine was told she could have up to two drinks per day! It's not worth the risk and it's really not a long time to be alcohol-free in the grand scheme of things.

Caffeine use over 200mg per day has been linked to miscarriages, and in very high quantities stillbirths. Caffeine is a stimulant and will cross the placenta to a growing baby, and similar to alcohol, caffeine needs to be metabolized by the liver—and in a baby's case, an immature one. For a pregnant woman, the ability to metabolize caffeine is also reduced as a pregnancy progresses, with double the time in the second trimester, and triple the time in the third trimester. A popular addition to smoothies is chocolate, and in alternative health circles the use of raw cacao. Raw cacao is more nutritious but both contain theobromine, not caffeine. Theobromine is still a stimulant and is still metabolized in the liver. One of the substances caffeine is broken down into is theobromine, so it's one step along the metabolic chain. Cacao is not considered problematic to nutrition like caffeine can be, but be mindful that if consuming raw cacao or dark chocolate with a high percentage of cocoa and it stimulates you, it will be stimulating your baby. Same thing will happen with breastfeeding. So it's best to limit or abstain from stimulating levels of cacao/chocolate during these times.

During preconception, you and your partner are both responsible for creating excellent quality egg and sperm, and should both be making the necessary changes. Once your pregnancy is "official," namely, past 13 weeks (or longer if needing further investigations such as an amniocentesis), Dad is off the hook! But let's hope he continues at least some of the good habits formed during the preconception period, as that will be best for his health in the long run. Then you are responsible for two—your health and well-being and that of your growing baby, particularly in the first and last trimesters. By 13 weeks your baby is fully formed and in the last trimester, many nutrients are transferred from mother to baby.

Dealing with Symptoms of Pregnancy

For many, the first signs of pregnancy arrive before the first missed menstrual period. Google "early pregnancy symptoms" and the lists are endless, with many signs similar to premenstrual symptoms, which makes things confusing and unreliable. Many women "just know" and the pregnancy test confirms what is suspected. After years of failed pregnancy tests, when I finally was pregnant, I knew it. I didn't usually experience much in the way of premenstrual symptoms, but around 1 week post-ovulation for a few days my boobs were very sore, and I was nauseous and insatiably thirsty. Below are some of the common symptoms of pregnancy and how to alleviate them.

NAUSEA AND HEARTBURN

Nausea in the first trimester is very common. According to my survey of smoothie-drinking mamas, 73 percent experienced nausea during pregnancy, 55 percent in the first trimester only, and an unlucky 12 percent all pregnancy. In addition, 33 percent described their nausea as moderately severe, 23 percent mild, and 17 percent severe.

Morning sickness or "emesis gravidarum," as its otherwise known, is considered to be due to the drop in blood sugar overnight and subsequent side effect of nausea in the morning; however, the majority of pregnant women do not have morning sickness in the morning! According to my survey, nausea with or without vomiting was reported as being in the morning, day, evening, all day, or no pattern—all with similar frequency.

Most common in the second half of pregnancy is heartburn. During pregnancy, the placenta releases progesterone (and levels continue to rise), which relaxes smooth muscles including the uterus, and also the valve at the top of the stomach, allowing stomach acids to flow into the esophagus and cause that unpleasant burning sensation in the chest. As baby gets bigger in late pregnancy, stomach acids can also be pushed into the esophagus due to the abdominal cavity being crowded. Variations in symptoms between women will hence be reliant on hormone levels and size and position of the baby/babies.

Personally, I always woke up feeling great in the morning of my pregnancy, but around mid-morning I started to feel queasy. Then by mid-afternoon (exactly 2:30 every day) it ramped up a notch and it was downhill from there. My last 3 hours of work were difficult and I was pretty useless all evening till bedtime. I only vomited twice but the almost constant nausea was very unsettling—like being hungover for 3 months! Heartburn then started in the 24th week and came and went for a while before being almost constant in the last 6 or so weeks. I didn't find food or smoothies relieving for either nausea or heartburn, and anything hot or spicy or sour was aggravating, so I only gained 11 pounds all pregnancy and lost weight over two occasions, as it was difficult to eat normally.

I had the worst morning sickness with my first, as I knew nothing of nutrition back then. I was just sick all day every day for around 2 months. I couldn't go in a car without vomiting. With my second it was much milder as my overall diet was better. By the time I got to my third I was much more aware, and found that small liquid meals like smoothies, more often, were helpful with the nausea. —Monica

Theories of Pregnancy Sickness

Reasons for nausea during pregnancy are not clear and can be
a bit contradictory. Some sources claim that a well-nourished
mother is less likely to have significant sickness. But it is also
said that sickness is a good sign of a healthy pregnancy, with
miscarriage more likely with little to no nausea experienced; yet
miscarriage is more common in poorly nourished mothers. Some
women report that their health was a clear factor, and others
not. More specifically, theories for why pregnancy sickness occurs
include:

- Rapid rise of HCG (human chorionic gonadotropin—a
  hormone that helps maintain pregnancy before the placenta
  matures) in early pregnancy. HCG starts to lower from around
  10 weeks as progesterone and estrogen continue to rise, so
  this can't explain sickness throughout pregnancy, as there are
  high levels of hormones generally all pregnancy

- A protective mechanism by the body to reduce the chances of
  the mother ingesting something potentially toxic to the baby

- Increased sensitivity and slowing down of the gastrointestinal
  tract (due to high progesterone) and change to olfactory
  centers, giving some women a "sensitive" stomach and/or
  problem with odors such as strong food smells or perfumes

- Genetic predisposition with greater chance of nausea if your
  mother experienced pregnancy sickness, too

- If carrying a girl, 50 percent more likely

- More likely if carrying multiples (due to extra hormones and
  extra space invading)

- Associated with a history of migraine or motion sickness

- Stress and fatigue—physical or mental

- Need for extra B6 and/or magnesium (both associated with stress, migraines, and motion sickness)
- Not enough protein due to the negative effect on blood sugar
- Developing gestational diabetes
- Dehydration—it can be double-edged sword when it's hard to keep fluids down!

For those who experience nausea and vomiting, the range of aggravating and easing factors does vary widely, with some women needing to eat frequently, while others can barely eat. According to my survey, there was no overwhelming tendency for food, drinks, or smoothies to relieve or stir up symptoms. The most common aggravating factors were spicy foods, dairy, fatty foods, sugary/sweet foods, and citrus. Protein, carbs, salty foods, water, and cool food/liquids were the ones that relieved the most, with bananas on the fence, leaning toward easing. For 38 percent of respondents, no foods/liquids aggravated symptoms, and for an unlucky 16 percent, nothing was relieving.

What helped my nausea in the first trimester aggravated my heartburn in the third—namely, orange juice, ginger, and peppermint. Milk aggravated nausea but helped my heartburn. What helped both was sipping cool water often, and I needed to design my morning smoothies rather carefully!

I had intense nausea throughout my second pregnancy. What helped were ice-cold smoothies and frozen fruit, especially grapes and bananas. —Bronwyn

Changing Your Smoothie Content While Pregnant

If your pregnancy was unplanned, or planned with minimal, if any, dietary changes, then being aware of nutritional needs and boosting the content of your smoothies will be of benefit. When moving from a preconception program such as outlined in Chapter 3, "Making Babies," recipes high in the desired nutrients for fertility are also good for pregnancy. However, ingredients like raw eggs should not be used, and sudden high usage of microalgae like spirulina or chlorella should be avoided due to the chances of triggering a detox reaction. For similar reasons, sudden planned changes in eating habits are not advised while pregnant, like quitting sugar, elimination diets, stopping all carbs, fad diets, doing a juice fast, etc. Generally, eating more healthily is perfectly fine, however! Feeling sick can suddenly change your eating habits, but this is largely out of your control.

Of the smoothie-drinking women in my survey, 37 percent changed their smoothie recipes when moving from usual smoothies to pregnancy smoothies. Reasons for the change were reactions to cravings, reactions to sickness, disallowed foods such as raw eggs, or extra nutritional demands. Low zinc can be associated with abnormal cravings in early pregnancy; hence, zinc-rich smoothies are an excellent idea.

Personally, I found my smoothies needed to be simple during my pregnancy: not too many ingredients and not too rich. I craved freshly squeezed orange juice in the first 2 months. A girlfriend of mine craved fats and did well on smoothies with a high fat content. Some women crave nothing and others can crave anything and everything! What was consistent between my friend and me, however, was the need to drink our smoothies slowly. I would take mine to work and sip it over a couple of hours. For a while I thought smoothies at breakfast time were making me nauseous, as my sickness would start mid-morning, so I tried non-smoothie breakfasts and different smoothie ingredients combos, particularly non-banana-based ones and non-green ones. But it was the same every day regardless. By 14 weeks I was okay with any morning smoothie again, though I preferred high-water-content fruits such as melons, or banana-based smoothies.

CONSTIPATION

One of the side effects of high levels of progesterone during pregnancy is slowing of the digestive process; hence, constipation can be a problem for pregnant women. Progesterone rises over the second half of the menstrual cycle and continues to rise as the pregnancy progresses, with associated increasing tendency toward constipation.

It is in the second half of pregnancy that constipation common, with rising progesterone and a growing baby pressing on the bowel. Combine this with poor fiber or fluid intake and little exercise, then getting backed up is very common. The solutions? Regular plant-based fiber is recommended, particularly soluble fiber, which is gentler to the gut. Soluble fiber forms a gel that is soothing to the gut and slows the emptying of food from the stomach to the small intestine, which is also good for blood sugar control, as it slows the dump of glucose to the blood. This assistance to control blood sugar may also help reduce symptoms of nausea. Also, ensure you are consuming at least eight glasses of water daily, and perform gentle, regular exercises such as walking, yoga, or Pilates.

Hemorrhoids

A complication of constipation may be hemorrhoids (though they may develop independently of constipation), so in addition to the suggestions listed, it is really important to avoid straining when using your bowel. Elevating your knees above hip height with your feet on a footrest when on the toilet can help by aligning the anus and rectum for easier defecation—similar to traditional squatting poses used for this purpose. This can get tricky when heavily pregnant, but should be manageable with the legs parted. Don't try this if suffering with significant pelvic instability, however.

Smoothie-friendly soluble sources of fiber: pears, blueberries, chia, apples, oranges, cucumber, celery, strawberries, mango, and plums

MOOD

Many women experience mood swings during pregnancy, some severe, where it's hard for family, close friends, and co-workers to relate to and cope with the pregnant woman in question. For many it's mild, with the odd cry over nothing in particular. The best strategies with significant mood problems is to acknowledge its happening, talk over feelings—especially with your partner—rest more if you are overdoing things, which may be overwhelming you, and seek medical help if your moods are very disruptive and if you are in a dark place. Depression can affect women while pregnant, and nutritionally this can be assisted by boosting intake of zinc, the amino acids tyrosine and tryptophan, vitamin C, B vitamins, magnesium, and essential fats, particularly omega-3 EPA and DHA. I had a very stressful pregnancy due to problems with my baby; however, I found my moods were surprisingly stable other than the odd moments of bursting into tears!

Smoothie- and pregnancy-friendly mood-boosting sources: leafy greens, avocado, peanuts, beets, almonds, dairy milk and yogurt, sunflower seeds, pumpkin seeds, pumpkin, sweet potato, carrots, fresh fruits (especially banana, citrus, and berries), chia seeds, beets, oats, and cacao

FLEXIBILITY AND INSTABILITY

Another hormone called relaxin, which is produced by the placenta, is responsible for increasing the flexibility of your soft tissues, namely ligaments (connective tissues that join bones together). Collagen is in connective tissue, and relaxin alters collagen metabolism by slowing its synthesis and increasing its breakdown, effectively making it looser. This makes the usually stiff joints of the pelvis somewhat flexible in preparation for birth, where the baby needs to travel from the abdomen to the outside world via the pelvis.

An unfortunate effect of relaxin in some women is suffering with instability, as their collagen becomes very loose and pelvis very unstable, causing pain and dysfunction. In my job as a physiotherapist I see this often. Frequently, it starts in the second trimester. With postural and movement-based advice, including performing pelvic-floor exercises, for many, symptoms of pelvic pain settle down, but for some they get worse, requiring compression belts to be worn around the hips and in some cases crutches to help walk.

Relaxin also softens or "ripens" the cervix and relaxes the muscular walls of the uterus, allowing them to stretch as baby grows. Relaxin also mediates change to the vascular system; with blood volume increasing by 50 percent, relaxin assists the organs and blood vessels of the body, including the heart and kidneys, to cope with this demand. There is nothing you can do about the release of relaxin into your system, though avoiding excessive weight-gain during pregnancy or avoiding heading into pregnancy overweight or obese is wise, as this may put more strain on loosening joints. I have always been a bit on the stiff side, so it was fortunate that the effect of relaxin on my system was the bonus of flexibility I don't usually have. I could touch my toes and my back felt great!

SKIN CARE

There are many reasons why your skin quality may change when not pregnant, including hormones, hydration, diet, hygiene, and exposure to sun or air conditioning. During pregnancy, however, you can bet any changes are due to your hormones, which encourage greater production of oil—perhaps why there is that "pregnancy glow" as skin is more plump and shiny. For some, this increase in oil production brings or worsens acne, and for others, skin quality improves. My skin has always been prone to spots, and I wasn't looking forward to how my skin would react while pregnant; however, I was really fortunate that my skin cleared up and literally glowed, pimple-free.

You can't alter the amount of pregnancy hormones in your system, but there are things you can do if your skin has erupted. Adele McConnell, creator of www.vegiehead.com, is a qualified beauty therapist, incredible plant-based cook, and has the most amazing glowing skin. Her top pregnancy skin-care tips are: *"Don't pick or squeeze pimples, as tempting as it is, and avoid touching your face generally. Cleanse, tone, and moisturize morning and night, cleanse twice if wearing makeup, avoid alcohol-based toners, and seek out natural skin care products. Changing your pillow slip [case] and face washer daily is also a good idea. Drink at least eight glasses of water every day, and eat a diet rich in good fats, the antioxidant vitamins A, C, and E, plus biotin, silica, and zinc."*

Biotin is also known as vitamin H or B7. Smoothie-friendly sources are milk and egg yolk; however, egg shouldn't be used in smoothies while pregnant. If you eat eggs, eat them regularly, cooked, for extra biotin. Silica is a trace mineral found in bones, hair, skin, and fingernails. It is a major building block of collagen, which helps keep skin supple.

Smoothie-friendly ingredients for healthy pregnant skin: nuts such as almonds, cashews, and macadamias; seeds such as chia, hemp, sunflower, and pumpkin; dairy milk and yogurt, leafy greens, avocado, coconut, oats, tahini, bananas, peanuts, beets, cucumber, cacao, maple syrup, carrots, pumpkin, sweet potato, and a variety of fresh colorful fruits

STRETCH MARKS

The other pressing skin concern of pregnancy is stretch marks! Also known as "striae gravidarum," these can occur anywhere there is rapid growth, namely the breasts and belly, but may also affect the lower back, hips, and thighs. Stretch marks are caused by tearing of the dermis or middle layer of the skin. Multiple factors are thought to influence their development, including weight gain greater than 30 pounds, hormones (relaxin, estrogen, cortisol), genetics, diet, hydration, larger baby weight, weight before pregnant, consuming caffeine or alcohol, and age. So if you are an obese teenager who puts on more than 30 pounds, has a big baby, has poor nutrition, is dehydrated, and your mother got stretch marks, you will very likely get them, too! The application of topical lotions can be quite an obsession for many women, but there is little to no evidence to support their use. Nutritionally, the best things for skin elasticity are the same nutrients as described for managing acne: vitamins A, C, and E, plus biotin, silica, and zinc.

My sister and I were pregnant at the same time. I was fortunate not to get stretch marks but she did, so that throws genetics out the window. However, she had a much bigger baby, was 10 days overdue, and she put on more weight than I did, so it's likely no surprise that size is a big factor in over-stretching the skin.

Smoothie-friendly ingredients for pregnancy stretch-mark prevention: nuts such as almonds, cashews, and macadamias; seeds such as chia, hemp, sunflower, and pumpkin; dairy milk and yogurt, leafy greens, avocado, coconut, oats, tahini, bananas, peanuts, beets, cucumber, cacao, maple syrup, carrots, pumpkin, sweet potato, and a variety of fresh colorful fruits

SWELLING

Due to the 50 percent increase in blood volume, and because the body hangs onto extra sodium due to pregnancy hormones, swelling of the extremities occurs in the majority of pregnant women. This is particularly in the lower limbs, which in combination with relaxin hormone softening ligaments of the feet can result in a half or full size bigger shoe. Swelling can also affect the hands, making wearing rings difficult. Nutritionally, the most important thing is to stay well hydrated—reducing fluid can make swelling worse as the body feels it needs to hang onto fluid to stay hydrated. Swelling of course will worsen with gravity and improve with rest and elevation, so most women find lower limb swelling is largely gone each morning.

Additionally, too little or too much sodium can be a problem for fluid balance, so use good-quality mineral salt to taste, but avoid heavily salted, processed and junk foods that are very high in poor-quality salt. Increasing potassium-rich fruit and vegetables can also help balance sodium, and using a smoothie as a meal or snack means you will get a nice serving of fluid to help stay hydrated.

Smoothie-friendly ingredients for managing pregnancy fluid retention: water, coconut water, cucumbers, melons, nuts, and seeds (especially pumpkin seeds, hemp seeds, chia seeds, and tahini), raw cacao, leafy greens (such as spinach, mint, beet leaves, Swiss chard, and kale), beets, blackberries, raspberries, quinoa, oats, bananas, yogurt, dried apricots, dried peaches, avocado, and figs

BLOOD PRESSURE

Raised blood pressure is common, particularly if the mother is stressed or nervous, which can easily happen at a doctor's office when your blood pressure is tested. A number of times my blood pressure was raised, probably due to the stress of knowing my baby had a birth defect, but it didn't help as I was then worried my blood pressure would be raised when tested (as it inevitably was)! If it was retested after a few minutes of doing some relaxing breathing it usually went down and I had no other symptoms of concern.

For others, blood pressure can lower, which starts in early pregnancy and peaks in the second trimester as a result of the expansion of blood volume and relaxation of blood vessel walls. Typical symptoms are dizziness, which can lead to fainting, particularly when getting up too quickly or standing still for too long.

If swelling occurs in the hands and face, a considerable amount of weight is gained quickly, and if there are headaches or vision disturbances, you may have preeclampsia, a serious condition for the mother and the baby that needs immediate medical assessment and attention. High blood pressure and protein in the urine will confirm the diagnosis. The "eclampsia" part of preeclampsia refers to seizures, which is what can happen if it's not treated. Preeclampsia is a problem that stems from abnormal blood flow through the placenta and is associated most with women who are obese; of black race; have insulin resistance; have high homocysteine; have high blood pressure, diabetes, or kidney disease (prenatally); are carrying multiple babies; are a teen mother or over 40; and/or have a thrombophilic disorder (excessive blood clotting).

Considered to be as common as 8 to 10 percent of pregnancies, the more severe cases tend to result in premature birth via induction or C-section. Naturally, many of these risk factors are unavoidable; however, planning for pregnancy can involve reduction of risk factors, such as losing weight (which may in turn normalize blood pressure and insulin resistance if those are issues). If homocysteine is high, then lowering strategies can be implemented via a diet rich in "methyl group" donors such as methylated B vitamins, choline, betaine, zinc, and magnesium. (For more on methylation and homocysteine see Chapter 3, "Making Babies.")

Smoothie-friendly ingredients for cardiovascular health during pregnancy: leafy greens (such as spinach, cruciferous vegetables, parsley, cilantro, and mint); sunflower and chia seeds, beets, goji berries, bananas, peanuts, oats, sweet potato, pumpkin, raw cacao, avocado, dairy milk, and yogurt

WEIGHT GAIN

Obesity has risen significantly over the past 20 years. About 52 percent of Australian women are overweight or obese, and in the United States it's 64 percent. The prevalence of obesity in pregnancy is also rising, which is problematic because of the link to increased complications of labor and delivery, such as gestational diabetes and/or preeclampsia. Maternal obesity also slows dilation of the cervix, increasing the risk of prolonged labor and interventions such as inductions and caesarean sections. Moreover, risks to babies include still birth, lower APGAR (appearance, pulse, grimace, activity, respiration) scores immediately post-birth, and large weight, and babies are more likely to be admitted to special care. Complications are most common with already obese women who gain excessive weight, versus small to moderate gains while obese, or large gains if of an average to overweight frame. Underweight women and obese women are less likely to gain excessively versus average weight to overweight women. Guidelines updated and published by the Institute of Medicine (IOM) in 2009 specified recommended weight gain per category of body mass index (BMI), suggesting that:

- Underweight women with a BMI of less than 18.5 may gain between 28 and 40 pounds (12.5kg to18kg).

- Normal weight women with a BMI of 18.5 to 24.9 may gain between 25 and 35 pounds (11.5kg to 16kg).

- Overweight women with a BMI of 25 to 29.9 may gain between 15 and 25 pounds (7kg to 11.5kg).

- Obese women with a BMI over 30 may gain between 11 and 20 pounds (5kg to 9kg).

Note: BMI is calculated by dividing weight in kilograms by height in meters squared—for instance, 70(kg) divided by 1.7(m)² equals a BMI of 24, which is normal. In standard, it is weight in pounds divided by height in inches squared, and then the total is multiplied by 703.

When weight gains are within these ranges, it has been found that this results in the best outcomes for mothers and babies. However, the weight gain by most pregnant women is out of these ranges. Furthermore, it has been found that regularly weighing pregnant women or not has little to no bearing on their weight gain and health outcomes. This may simply highlight that women cannot easily control their appetite once pregnant—particularly when it comes to dealing with nausea. It is reported that up to 70 percent of pregnant women gain excess weight, which is similar to the prevalence of pregnant women reporting sickness. Studies looking at dietary interventions while pregnant, such as dietary counseling, diets, and exercises, have not revealed any consistent findings, except that women on a low-glycemic diet plus exercise during pregnancy are most likely to be successful managing pregnancy weight.

If excessive weight gain during pregnancy is an issue for you, or is likely to be based on previous experience, then aiming to enter pregnancy with a healthy weight is the best course of action. Both before and during pregnancy, aiming to exercise three to four times weekly (gentler forms during pregnancy, are best) and eating a diet and drinking smoothies with a low glycemic load should be the goal. Unless you are loading up your smoothies with extra sweeteners, most smoothies can be considered low glycemic; however, very sweet fruits such as mangoes, grapes, and bananas are the ones to limit, as they have a higher glycemic load. On the other hand, if these fruits happen to be the ones that alleviate your nausea, eat them anyway!

GESTATIONAL DIABETES

The diagnosis of gestational diabetes mellitus (GDM) is when high blood glucose levels first develop during pregnancy. It is estimated that 3 to 8 percent of pregnant women develop GDM usually between the 24th and 28th weeks, thus contributing to excessive weight gain during pregnancy for the mother and baby. Maternal blood glucose levels usually return to normal after the birth; however, there is increased risk for the mother and child to develop type 2 diabetes in the future. It also increases the risk of preterm delivery via C-section due to the baby's large size.

Pregnant women are most likely to get GDM if they are over 30 years old, are overweight or obese leading into pregnancy, gain weight excessively during pregnancy—especially the first trimester—have a family history of diabetes, have had GDM in a previous pregnancy, and/or have backgrounds that include indigenous Australians, Torres Strait Islanders, Polynesians, Melanesians, Vietnamese, Chinese, or Middle Eastern.

Hence, the main risk-management strategy is to aim to enter pregnancy with a healthy weight, as discussed in the previous section.

I was diagnosed with gestational diabetes (GDM) while pregnant and found I could tweak my smoothie recipes to include less of the ingredients that would spike my blood glucose and more of the slow-release carbohydrates. I have a bit of a sweet tooth, despite my best efforts to curb it, so instead of adding honey or maple syrup to my smoothie I would add a date or just vanilla, so I would have a bit of a sweet flavor without having to worry about my blood glucose levels. —Serena

URINARY FREQUENCY

During the first trimester of pregnancy, high HCG increases blood flow to pelvic organs and stimulates the kidneys to eliminate waste more quickly, resulting in the need to pee rather frequently! This settles during the second trimester, due to HCG lowering as the placenta takes over hormonal control of the pregnancy. During the third trimester, the baby is taking up much more room and does a great job at compressing the bladder, increasing frequency once again. If you have a weak pelvic floor from a previous pregnancy, urinary frequency will likely be significant, so don't forget your pelvic floor exercises. However, don't be tempted to reduce fluid intake to avoid peeing so often, because you need to be well hydrated.

CRAMPS

Many systems in the human body rely on the amount of, and balance between, the minerals magnesium and calcium, and potassium and sodium. This includes the issue of blood pressure and also affects muscle tone. Cramping muscles, especially for the lower legs, are a common symptom of pregnancy, reported by 30 to 50 percent of pregnant women. Most notably these painful muscle spasms affect the large calf muscles but can affect others too, and usually overnight. If not cramps, you may experience restless legs when trying to get to sleep. The need for more potassium, calcium, and magnesium is generally required.

I remember getting increasingly uncomfortable legs in the evenings as my pregnancy progressed in the latter half. I also worked largely on my feet up until 3 weeks before the birth of my daughter. What helped was stretching my calves, massages, keeping well hydrated, and days with less weight-bearing. I ensured my smoothies and diet generally were magnesium-, calcium-, and potassium-rich, and I also took a calcium/magnesium powder before bed——if I didn't I was guaranteed a wicked cramp overnight!

Smoothie-friendly ingredients to combat cramps during pregnancy: dairy milk and yogurt, almonds and almond milk, seeds (such as pumpkin, hemp, and chia), quinoa, tahini, leafy greens (such as spinach, beet leaves, mint, Swiss chard, and kale), raspberries, blackberries, oats, bananas, and figs

FATIGUE

The first trimester of pregnancy is very tiring! Your body is undergoing huge changes, including rising hormones, increased blood volume, and growing a placenta—your baby's lifeline! The second trimester is when most women feel their best, certainly when it comes to energy levels. By the time the third trimester arrives and progresses, fatigue again sets in as you are carrying around a lot more weight, and nutrients such as iron are transferred to the baby from your stores, which can also contribute to feeling tired if iron levels, particularly if iron stores (ferritin) become low (see the "Iron" section in this chapter for more about iron).

Apart from rest, nutrition can play an important role. More frequent smaller meals can help with maintaining blood sugar, which is harder while pregnant. Additionally, protein at each meal can help with blood sugar control. Good-quality carbohydrates, such as those found in fruits, and good-quality fats also help to maintain energy.

In the final trimester, particularly if iron is low, focusing on iron-rich foods eaten in combination with vitamin C–rich foods to aid absorption is essential. Smoothies are an excellent way to get all of these ingredients in one easy-to-prepare package. Fruits provide carbohydrate and vitamin C; leafy greens if used provide iron and protein; nuts and seeds provide fats and protein; and avocado and coconut products provide fabulous fats and fiber. And because it's not uncommon for pregnant women to struggle with large portions and do better with more frequent eating, smoothies can be sipped over a few hours if need be or easily portioned (i.e., half for breakfast and half for a mid-morning snack).

The main reason I love smoothies is for the convenience. I love that I can just pop it all in the blender, whiz it up, and in a few minutes have a smoothie in a cup ready to sip on the way to work. It was easier for me to manage that way, especially during the early weeks of the pregnancy when I felt nauseated in the morning. During my pregnancy I became quite iron depleted, so smoothies were a great way for me to be able to add iron-rich vegetables to my diet without feeling like I was eating mountains of green leafy veggies. —Leanne

Nutrients Essential to a Pregnant Mother

VITAMINS AND MINERALS ESSENTIAL TO A PREGNANT MOTHER

Nutrients needed during pregnancy are similar to the nutrients needed for a couple trying to conceive. Here I have highlighted the differences and which nutrients help which functions. If you would like a more thorough reading on the nutrients, see Chapter 3, "Making Babies."

Iron

Iron is needed for the formation of red blood cells, which carry oxygen around the body to all tissues, including to a growing baby. Maternal blood volume increases by 50 percent during pregnancy, and iron is essential for rapidly growing and differentiating cells. Severe iron deficiency poses a risk to the development of a baby's blood supply, organs (especially the brain), and iron stores after birth. However, nutritionally the baby will take priority and receive adequate iron, leaving Mama-to-be rather tired as she becomes more iron deficient. Even women with good iron stores prenatally and during pregnancy can find themselves iron deficient in the third trimester, as the transfer of iron from the mother's stores to the baby's stores increases, and it doubles in the last few weeks of gestation.

As discussed in Chapter 3, heme iron, which comes from animal sources, is more easily absorbed than non-heme iron found from plants. In smoothies, heme iron sources are limited in pregnancy as raw eggs are out, and dairy is a poor source.

Iron is the main nutrient linked to anemia; however, other B vitamins, namely folate, B12, and B6, are all important for red blood cell health and all can contribute to an anemic state, which by definition is a lack of red blood cells or hemoglobin (the iron-continuing protein) by number or quality. There are over 400 types of anemia, which are divided into three categories according to cause: loss of blood, reduced or abnormal red blood cell production, and destruction of red blood cells. Short of an inherited condition like sickle cell anemia, it will most likely be nutrient deficiency that is the problem during pregnancy.

Smoothie-friendly iron sources for pregnancy: leafy greens, especially spinach, chard, and parsley; dried apricots, figs, raspberries, raisins, prunes, beets, raw cacao, tahini, turmeric, pumpkin seeds, hemp seeds, chia seeds, and quinoa

Vitamin A
During pregnancy, this antioxidant and fat-soluble vitamin is important for the immune system, skin, and lungs, given they all get quite a workout! For baby, vitamin A is necessary for organ development such as the lungs, kidneys, and heart. It is also essential for facilitating communication between the sense organs and the brain, notably for vision and hearing. Vitamin A deficiency is rare in the developed world, but it is one of the top causes of

preventable blindness in children and xerophthalmia (a severe and progressive eye disease) in pregnant women, with early signs that include night blindness and inability to see in low light. With regard to immunity, vitamin A deficiency increases the severity and mortality risk of infections, particularly diarrhea and measles. A deficiency of vitamin A has also been linked to the development of cleft palate deformities.

As discussed in Chapter 3, preformed vitamin A (retinol) from animals is more easily assimilated than carotenoids in plants. So if not enough retinol is being consumed, then carotenoids will be utilized to top it up.

Smoothie-friendly beta-carotene sources for pregnancy: yellow/orange/red fruits and leafy greens, especially carrots, pumpkin, sweet potato, spinach, kale, cantaloupe, mango, papaya, passion fruit, apricots, peaches, nectarines, and kiwi

B Vitamins

The B-group vitamins include B1, B2, B3, B5, B6, B9 (folate), B12, biotin, and choline. All of the B vitamins work together to help create blood cells for a growing baby. They are important for brain development, cell division, and energy production, and they assist a baby to reach a healthy birth weight and reduce the incidence of birth defects. They also help to boost progesterone (particularly B6), which continues to rise until the end of a pregnancy. Biotin, as we discussed earlier, is good for skin and hair.

All B vitamins work with the minerals magnesium and manganese. Manganese is available in cinnamon, passion fruit, strawberries, turmeric, oats, sweet potato, kiwi, beets, and leafy greens, especially spinach and brassicas. The best source is pineapple, but for many pregnant women pineapple is too acidic in smoothies and may cause nausea or heartburn.

The importance of folate and B12 was discussed in detail in Chapter 3, with regard to fertility and the prevention of neural tube defects. In summary, vitamin B12 is important for thyroid function, mood, healthy blood, the nervous system, detoxification, reduction of homocysteine, and hormone balance. Folate is also important for healthy blood, the nervous system, reducing homocysteine, mood, and is of paramount important for new cell production—particularly when growing a new human!

Folate and B12 are important for good health irrespective of pregnancy, but their need is greater in the first trimester, and given 50 percent of pregnancies are unplanned, it's especially important that women of childbearing years not be deficient. A baby's organs are all formed by the end of the first trimester and the neural tube starts to close around 6 weeks (4 weeks post-conception). Folate, B12, and choline are all necessary to ensure the neural tube closes properly, and if it doesn't, it risks the development of disabling spina bifida or fatal anencephaly. Even with a diet replete with sources of folate, all women planning to get pregnant and during the first trimester are advised to take a folate supplement of at least 400mcg and ensure the diet is rich in choline and B12 at the same time—or supplement B12 if it is known to be low.

Smoothie- and pregnancy-friendly B vitamin sources:

B1: macadamias, sunflower seeds, sweet potato, chia, cilantro, oats, peanuts, and beet greens

B2: almonds, spinach, sweet potato, pumpkin, beet greens, mint, collards, maple syrup, milk, and yogurt

B3: peanuts, sunflower seeds, sweet potato, chia, and avocado

B5: avocado, sunflower seeds, sweet potato, strawberries, yogurt, and peanuts

B6: avocado, bananas, carrots, leafy greens (especially spinach, kale, and collards), fennel, prunes, dried apricots, sweet potato, beets, and sunflower seeds

Folate: leafy greens, especially spinach, collards, kale, parsley, and romaine lettuce; avocado, peanuts, beets, oranges, papaya, mangoes, banana, sunflower seeds, walnuts, and cantaloupe

B12: dairy milk and yogurt

Choline: sunflower seeds, pumpkin, peanuts

Eggs are a great source of B vitamins, but raw eggs should not be used in smoothies for pregnancy.

Vitamin C

For the mother-to-be, vitamin C has a role to play with the development (or not) of stretch marks and provides strength to the amniotic sac. Vitamin C is also necessary for the production of reproductive hormones that are higher during pregnancy, particularly progesterone, which continues to rise over the full term of pregnancy.

It is also essential for the function of osteoblasts, which are cells that produce new hard bone—this is particularly important for the development of baby's bones and teeth in partnership with vitamin D and calcium. Vitamin C cannot be stored and must be supplied daily.

Smoothie- and pregnancy-friendly vitamin C sources: Abundant in fruit and vegetables, particularly brassicas (or cruciferous vegetables), parsley, papaya, avocado, passion fruit, beets, pomegranates, strawberries, mangoes, bananas, kiwi, citrus, and melons. Vitamin C also complements the action of antioxidant phytochemicals such as bioflavonoids, which are abundant in citrus and tropical fruit, and anthocyanins, which are color pigments found in berries, cherries, grapes, plums, and bananas.

Vitamin D

Another fat-soluble vitamin, vitamin D works with calcium and phosphorus for the health of bones and teeth, including the formation of tooth enamel in the baby in utero. The rapid skeletal growth of the baby in the third trimester can tax the mother's stores, particularly if her intake of vitamins C and D plus calcium is inadequate. A significant deficiency in the mother is likely to lead to the baby being deficient at birth, risking the development of rickets.

Doses 10 times higher than the RDA of 400IU taken during pregnancy have been linked to a reduction in incidence of pregnancy complications, such as gestational diabetes, premature births, and infections, and such doses are considered safe. These doses of vitamin D require supplementation (under professional advice) and can't easily be met by diet. As discussed in Chapter 3, "Making Babies," if supplementing, be sure to get vitamin D3 and not vitamin D2. Meanwhile, ensure you get sun on your skin as often as you can without getting sunburned. The most smoothie-friendly dietary source is good-quality raw eggs—but not while pregnant.

Vitamin E

Tocopherol is another name of vitamin E, which is Greek in origin, with "tokos" meaning child/offspring and "pherein" meaning to bear/carry. It is an important nutrient for fertility and pregnancy and one of the least likely to be deficient in—unless you eat very few plant foods. Similar to vitamin C, vitamin E is an antioxidant vitamin, meaning it helps to fight free radical damage in the body and has a role to play in keeping skin supple and the amniotic sac strong.

Vitamin E is transferred from the mother to baby during the third trimester. It assists with the transport of oxygen to cells, and its antioxidant role helps to protect the RNA and DNA (our genetic code) from damage that may lead to birth defects.

Smoothie- and pregnancy-friendly vitamin E sources: leafy greens (especially chard and spinach), avocado, sunflower seeds, almonds, peanuts, mint, papaya, kiwi, nectarines, and raspberries

Vitamin K

Involved in the manufacture of prothrombin, vitamin K helps make blood clot. It is also important for bone health by ensuring calcium lays down into bone and not into soft tissues. Vitamin K1 is found in green leafy vegetables and vitamin K2 in the meat of grass-fed animal fats and fermented foods. K2 can also be manufactured by the conversion of K1 by gut bacteria. Both forms of vitamin K have similar functions in the body; however, K2 has greater cardiovascular protective properties, in addition to playing a more important role in maintaining bone density. Vitamin K, along with the other fat-soluble vitamins A, D, and E, doesn't cross the placenta as easily as the water-soluble B vitamins and vitamin C, so it is not as abundant in fetal circulation. Combine this with the fact that the baby's gut is sterile at birth and there is not much vitamin K in breast milk, and you have the reason why a vitamin K injection is offered for the baby immediately after birth to reduce the risk of bleeding, particularly in the brain.

Some parents choose not to have their infant injected with vitamin K; rather, the mother ensures she is consuming plentiful sources of vitamin K prenatally from green leafy vegetables, fermented foods, and grass-fed animal fats such as butter and milk. Vitamin K is also an important vitamin for a pregnant woman to consume because she doesn't want any issues with bleeding either! However, there are a number of conditions that can lead to vitamin K deficiency and there are also conditions that cause abnormal clotting. Given the complexity of this issue, it is important if you are not considering the vitamin K injection that you do your research and be guided by a trusted and appropriately experienced health professional.

Smoothie- and pregnancy-friendly vitamin K1 sources: leafy greens such as kale, spinach, collards, turnip greens, and parsley

Smoothie- and pregnancy-friendly vitamin K2 sources: milk from grass-fed dairy cows, and fermented beverages such as kombucha and kefir

Calcium

We know calcium is needed for healthy bones, teeth, and muscles in adults—and this goes for the needs of a growing baby too. As previously discussed, vitamin D is needed to utilize calcium and phosphorus, which must be balanced for good bone density. Phosphorus is not a common nutrient deficiency due to its relative abundance in foods; however, it can be negatively affected by the use of antacid medications, which are frequently used by pregnant women in the latter stages of pregnancy (a time when the bone-building minerals are most important for the baby's rapidly developing skeleton) for relief of heartburn.

....

Home Remedy Antacid

If suffering from heartburn and using antacids, you can instead try a teaspoon of slippery elm powder mixed with a quarter cup of milk or water (try shaking it in a small jar with a lid as it doesn't stir together well) and consume it before a meal and before bed. Drink immediately as it gets thick quickly—the mixture lines the esophagus, providing a barrier to acid reflux, and soothes an already irritated gut wall.

....

In order to supply sufficient calcium to the baby, calcium absorption from the intestines is raised by an increase in the circulating vitamin D3 levels, less calcium is excreted via urine than normal, and some calcium is acquired from the maternal skeleton. Reported loss of bone density during pregnancy is 3 percent (and 10 percent in teenagers), around 5 percent if breastfeeding for 6 months, and 10 percent for 12 months. This reduction in bone density returns to normal 3 to 6 months after weaning. Long term, the turnover of bone, due to pregnancy and lactation, may improve bone density, compared to women who have not had children or women that did not breastfeed. Some women who are significantly deficient to begin with, or have other relevant medical conditions, risk developing osteoporosis, which is a loss of at least 25 percent bone density. The drawing of calcium, it should be noted, is from the bones not the teeth; however, pregnancy can increase the risk of gingivitis (gum inflammation), which if not well managed may get infected and cause periodontal disease that can lead to tooth loss. I personally know a lady who this happened to after her last child, and she ended up having all of her teeth extracted and false teeth made, and she was only in her forties.

Because of these mechanisms in place to acquire extra calcium during pregnancy and lactation, there is no need to increase calcium consumption. Worldwide, the recommended daily allowance is 1g (1000mg) and a bit more for teenage or post-menopausal women.

Smoothie- and pregnancy-friendly calcium sources: leafy greens: ½ cup, 50mg to 100mg; dairy milk/calcium-enriched other milks (like rice milk): 1 cup/250ml, 300mg; yogurt: ¾ cup/175ml, 332mg; uncooked oats: 1 cup, 42mg; dried figs: 6–10 figs, 150mg; chia seeds: 2 tablespoons,177mg; almonds: ½ cup, 186mg; tahini: 2 tablespoons, 128mg

These are just smoothie-friendly sources of calcium. When looking at a diet as a whole, the addition of a wide variety of vegetables, greens, seaweeds, beans, and canned fish with bones (if not vegetarian) also provide plenty of calcium.

If making homemade almond milk using 1 cup of raw almonds to 1 liter of water, there will be approximately 93mg of calcium per cup of milk.

Chromium

Chromium is required for the digestion of fats, proteins, and carbohydrates, and there is greater need for chromium if the diet is high in simple sugars. In partnership with vitamin B3, chromium and certain amino acids form part of the glucose tolerance factor (GTF), which binds to insulin and enhances its effect threefold. Deficiency of this mineral is linked to digestive difficulties, insomnia, mood swings, fatigue, and blood sugar imbalances. These issues are all things common in pregnant women—even in the absence of pre-existing diabetes or the development of gestational diabetes. Hence, a diet that supplies chromium is essential and also may require supplementation under the guidance of a health professional.

Smoothie- and pregnancy-friendly chromium sources: oats, dairy milk, licorice, and apples. Depending on the source, cinnamon may or may not provide chromium. Either way, it is often used in conjunction with chromium to help stabilize blood sugar.

Iodine

Essential for a healthy pregnancy, iodine is needed to ensure that the thyroid functions optimally. Iodine is stored in the thyroid gland in small amounts, so it is needed from the diet regularly. Iodine (with the amino acid tyrosine) is needed to make the thyroid hormones T3 (triiodothyronine) and T4 (thyroxine). The number associated with T3 and T4 is the number of iodine atoms included in the structure of each hormone. The thyroid produces around 50 percent more thyroid hormones during pregnancy, and this can be seen with higher TSH (thyroid stimulating hormones) levels in the blood. These hormone changes should go back to normal postnatally; however, a breastfed baby relies on iodine from the mother, so both pregnant and lactating women should be consuming extra iodine.

The World Health Organization (WHO) recommends women who are pregnant or breastfeeding take 250µg of iodine, combining dietary sources and supplementation. The NHMRC in Australia recommends that women who are pregnant have 220µg of iodine per day, and when breastfeeding, 270µg per day.

The implication of iodine deficiency is an adverse effect on a baby's brain and nervous system development. Iodine deficiency is considered the most common preventable cause of mental retardation in the world. Iodized table salt has been a source of iodine since 1924 in the United States, in response to iodine deficiency in the food supply causing many cases of goiter (thyroid gland enlargement). However, this salt is manufactured sodium chloride and potassium iodide and tainted with processing chemicals. It is also not clear how much of the purported 250µg per half teaspoon is actually available at the time of consumption due to iodine's tendency to evaporate, and the questionable ability to fully utilize synthesized sources of iodine. Pure, naturally occurring salts are much better options, such as Himalayan crystal salts that contain 84 minerals and trace elements, including naturally occurring iodine, albeit less than iodized table salt. Sea salts are not recommended due to increasing pollution of the world's waterways, particularly in the Northern Hemisphere.

Neither natural nor synthesized salts are the most ideal sources of iodine. It is better to get it from food or good-quality supplements. The best sources of iodine are sea vegetables, oysters (160μg per 100g serving), sushi with seaweed (92μg per 100g serving), milk (32μg per 1 cup/250ml, yogurt (16μg per 100g serving), eggs (13μg per 60g egg), and strawberries (13 μg per cup/145g). The best sources, however, are at risk of heavy metal and pollution contamination (seaweeds, namely kelp), and oysters and sushi are out for pregnancy due to risk of food poisoning! Hence, you can see why authorities recommend supplementing.

Smoothie- and pregnancy-friendly iodine sources: milk, yogurt, and strawberries are the best options, but the amounts are not significant. Some folks like to add a pinch of dulse flakes to a smoothie, but the reality is it will provide very little nutrition in just a pinch, and larger amounts will be rather unpleasant.

Magnesium

As discussed in Chapter 3, "Making Babies," magnesium is particularly important for energy production, hormone balance, and it relaxes the nervous system. Deficiency lists are huge but examples of symptoms include irritability, headaches, dental problems, poor sleep, nausea, poor memory, muscle weakness, muscle twitches/cramps, constipation, blood sugar imbalance, and fatigue. Sounds a bit like pregnancy, doesn't it! Because a pregnant body works very hard, it needs more magnesium than usual for energy production, and magnesium is needed to help make genetic material (i.e., DNA) and for protein synthesis—hence, more is needed to build a baby.

For baby, magnesium also works with calcium and vitamin D to build bones and teeth, and is needed for the development of a healthy heart and muscular system. Magnesium, with vitamin B6, also ensures ongoing and rising progesterone production, which is necessary for a healthy pregnancy, as deficiency has been implicated with miscarriages.

Like zinc, magnesium is easily depleted in the presence of alcohol, caffeine, sugar, phytates, many prescription medications, and stress. Chocolate or cocoa/cacao is an excellent source of magnesium, but given most chocolate is high in sugar and cacao (particularly raw chocolate and other dark chocolate varieties), it can be quite stimulating from the theobromine content, so chocolate is not an ideal food during pregnancy, and certainly not in large quantities. Loading up a smoothie with lots of raw cacao is not a great idea. Be guided by how it makes you feel—if you are feeling stimulated then it will have that effect on the baby to some degree too.

Smoothie- and pregnancy-friendly magnesium sources: nuts and seeds, especially pumpkin seeds and tahini; raw cacao; leafy greens, such as spinach, mint, beet leaves, Swiss chard, and kale; beets, blackberries, raspberries, quinoa, oats, hemp seeds, chia seeds, bananas, and figs

Selenium

Pregnancy is demanding to the mother's body with regard to the amount of nutrients that need to be delivered to the growing baby via the placenta. There is greater oxidative stress as a result, so the need for extra antioxidants is very important. See page 54 for further reading on selenium.

Smoothie- and pregnancy-friendly selenium sources: Brazil nuts are the best source, and to a lesser extent sunflower seeds, cashews, macadamias, and oats.

Zinc

As explained on page 55, zinc has more than 300 biological functions in the human body. All of these roles are important whether you are pregnant or not, but of particular benefit to pregnancy is blood sugar balance, which can affect mood and sickness. Zinc is also important for prevention and management of postnatal depression. Insufficient zinc can lead to abnormal cravings during pregnancy, and if homocysteine levels are raised, there is greater risk of pregnancy complications such as pregnancy-induced hypertension, preeclampsia, bleeding, infections, and prolonged labor. Zinc deficiency is also associated with hair loss with thyroid dysfunction.

The development of the placenta during pregnancy is directly related to zinc levels in a woman's body, and the placenta is what nourishes the developing baby. Zinc is essential for all areas of a baby's growth, from successful fertilization to the development of the nervous system, brain, organs, bones, teeth, and hair, and for energy production. Zinc is also important for the baby to grow to a healthy weight, to deliver to term, and to avoid birth defects.

Zinc is easily depleted by caffeine and alcohol consumption, the contraceptive pill, copper, iron (particularly if supplementing and taking at the same time), and phytates from whole grains. Furthermore, if gluten intolerance is not well managed, the gut won't absorb zinc very well. Zinc is also a nutrient that isn't stored, so regular and ideally daily supply is needed—and most importantly during preconception and pregnancy.

Smoothie- and pregnancy-friendly zinc sources: raw cacao, chia seeds, coconut, cashews, Swiss chard, parsley, macadamias, maple syrup, oats, pecans, peanuts, hemp seeds, pumpkin seeds, tahini, figs, spinach, ginger root, almonds, and sunflower seeds

MACRONUTRIENTS ESSENTIAL TO A PREGNANT MOTHER

Fats

As discussed in Chapter 2, "Fabulous Fats," fats are essential to pregnancy. We need many types of fats for healthy cell function, to build hormones, and to absorb fat-soluble vitamins—the most important being saturated, monounsaturated, omega-3, and cholesterol. One of the hormones produced by the placenta is HCG, or human chorionic gonadotropin. HCG essentially keeps the corpus luteum (of the ovary that released the egg) producing progesterone until the placenta is able to do it on its own. HCG production begins as soon as implantation takes place and is what is tested for with pregnancy tests. HCG also functions to access energy and nutrients from maternal stored fat. We have three types of fat: Structural fats are in our cheeks, heels, and around our organs, which we don't want to lose; reserve fat is what the body can access for energy easily and is what is lost with usual weight loss programs; and stored fat is on our hips, thighs, stomach, arms, and includes cellulite. During the first trimester, when HCG is acting, it can access this stored fat as an energy source, if needed, for the changes that need to occur to grow a baby, such as breast growth, blood volume increase, and placental growth. If you have ever seen a pregnant woman who has had hyperemesis gravidarum (the most severe form of pregnancy sickness), you will notice she has a belly but her arms and legs look like sticks. This effect is rather useful if the mother-to-be is feeling rather unwell, as 70 percent of pregnant women are in the first third of pregnancy, and unable to eat enough to provide the energy her body needs. Like the preferential transfer of nutrients to the baby, it's the mother that suffers and not the baby most of the time.

Smoothie- and pregnancy-friendly fats: coconut flesh from drinking coconuts, coconut cream and milk, avocado, macadamia, chia, flax, hemp, and walnuts. Still nutritious, but not as useful when it comes to fats, are other nuts and seeds such as cashews, almonds, sunflower seeds, and pumpkin seeds. Raw eggs are omitted for pregnancy in smoothies, but eggs can be eaten regularly if well cooked.

••

Health Comes First

Leading up to my pregnancy I was largely a vegetarian, eating fish occasionally, eggs often, and little to no dairy (due to intolerance). I ate plenty of nuts, quinoa, chia, and hemp, but increasingly not a lot of grains or legumes as they didn't agree with my guts all too well. I felt I was getting adequate protein, but about halfway through my pregnancy I was craving roast chicken. I tried to fight it because I had not eaten meat in such a long time and felt that it was better for my health and ethically better not to eat meat. However, my diet had become more limited by my food intolerances and thyroid issues (no gluten, dairy, soy, or raw brassicas), and feeling sick as a result of pregnancy also limited the volumes I could eat. I had to listen to my body and I gave in, and I have to admit I felt better. I needed the protein, and as it turned out I needed more iron too—even though I had an iron-rich green smoothie every morning.

When making decisions about food, my belief is that health should be the driving force. At one time, being vegetarian was a choice I made primarily for my health, but as time went on and my choices from the plant kingdom became more limited, I had to be realistic about what I needed to eat to nourish my body. I am still not entirely comfortable with eating animals from a welfare point of view, but I choose to eat as ethically as possible, sourcing eggs and meat that are free range and organic, and where possible having knowledge of the farms they come from.

••

Protein

Required for growth and repair, protein is important to support the extra growth during pregnancy, including the extra blood being made and for growth tissues of the breast, uterus, placenta, and of course the baby! Protein is something that most people are not deficient in, particularly if meat, dairy, and eggs are eaten in the diet. A well-planned vegetarian or vegan diet will also supply more than enough protein, provided a balance of grains, legumes, and nuts are eaten to ensure that all amino acids (the building blocks of protein) are consumed. Grains, nuts, and seeds lack the amino acid lysine and legumes lack methionine; however, chia, buckwheat, soy, and quinoa are complete proteins from the plant kingdom, which means they contain all eight essential amino acids.

Looking at expert opinions such as the WHO, AAP in the United States, and the NHMRC in Australia, the recommendations are similar: 0.75g of protein per kilogram (0.34g per pound) of body weight is what a woman should aim for normally, and this rises to 1g (0.45g per pound) during the second and third trimesters of pregnancy and 1.1g (0.49g per pound) while breastfeeding.

Smoothie- and pregnancy-friendly proteins: leafy greens, nuts and seeds, peanuts, dairy milk and yogurt, and plant-based protein powders (Miessence or Amazonia brands are the best)

Having gone through IVF and being very fortunate to get pregnant at the first attempt, I knew it was time to step up my healthy lifestyle even further. My growing baby and my rapidly changing body needed as many nutrients as possible. I created a green smoothie off the top of my head one day and used ingredients that I already had in the house, including spinach, kale, avocado, yogurt, almonds, honey, chia seeds, and quinoa. I religiously drank variations of it every day of my pregnancy, and 2 years later I'm still drinking it as

I continue to breastfeed my 17-month-old daughter. I will likely drink it forever—it's part of our family ritual now! Even my husband drinks it, and though my daughter is not so sure yet, she will love it one day, I hope. —Vicky

Probiotics

As discussed in Chapter 3, "Making Babies," probiotics or, "friendly bacteria," are essential to gut health and immunity—for everyone. Probiotic consumption is highly recommended during pregnancy, and therefore some form of probiotic should ideally be taken daily. Probiotic supplements come in a liquid, powder, or capsule forms, making it very simple to add to any smoothie without affecting the taste or texture.

Pregnant women are more prone to colds due to being immunocompromised and frequently experience a plethora of digestive issues, including nausea, heartburn, bloating, gas, and constipation. The vagina is also more susceptible to developing thrush from candida overgrowth, due to higher levels of estrogen present.

Smoothie- and pregnancy-friendly probiotic sources: supplements in liquid, capsule, or powder forms; kefir (based on water, or coconut water or milk), natural yogurt, and kombucha

....

Thrush and Group B Strep

Thrush is a candida overgrowth condition that causes discomfort, itching, and abnormal discharge. If thrush exists during a vaginal birth, the baby will likely get oral thrush, which can then transfer to the breasts of the mother while breastfeeding. A candida infection in the breasts can be very painful and can make the task of establishing breastfeeding difficult. In this situation both baby and mother need to be treated, usually with topical antifungals to the baby's mouth and mother's nipples. The mother and baby will also benefit from probiotics internally, and the mother should avoid sugar and yeast in her diet. The same goes for trying to manage thrush during pregnancy.

With regard to smoothies, some believe that no fruit should be eaten when experiencing thrush, as its sugars will also feed the candida. Options with smoothies are to either have a break from them if they are always fruit-based ones, or make smoothies with the least sweet fruit such as berries and green apples. Another option is to make smoothies without fruit, such as those that are more savory, based on non-sweet fruits like cucumbers, and/or smoothies that contain probiotic-containing liquids, such as yogurt or kefir.

Another issue some women have is testing positive to a rectal or vaginal swab in the third trimester (usually between 35 and 37 weeks) for Group B Strep (GBS). This bacteria exists in the intestines and will colonize the vagina in 10 to 30 percent of pregnant women. GBS is generally considered harmless as it exists as described, but the risk is that a baby born vaginally may contract a serious infection such as a blood infection, pneumonia, or meningitis. The medical treatment of choice is to administer IV (intravenous) antibiotics during labor. Some women use natural therapies to treat the infection, such as probiotics, vitamin C, and garlic, and may retest as negative in the hope they can avoid the antibiotics. The reason antibiotics are not given to treat GBS when it's found is that it can come back again. However, if a urinary tract infection (UTI) is positive for GBS during pregnancy, antibiotics are given and these mothers will have the IV during labor without a swab even being done, as will any mother who had GBS in a previous pregnancy. The exception is if a caesarean section is done before any waters break. Medical professionals are unlikely to support a natural approach only to dealing with GBS, but even if IV antibiotics go ahead and you have used extra probiotics, these will do no harm and will likely be better for your ability to cope with being treated with antibiotics.

Smoothies for Pregnant Mothers

According to my survey, 63 percent of women drinking smoothies while pregnant and breastfeeding did not change the content of their smoothie compared to their usual pre-pregnancy recipes. Given nutrient requirements are different and more demanding during these times, it is wise to make smoothies more nutritious than usual, particularly if the typical smoothie is just milk and a banana—not that this isn't nutritious, but it can be better.

If thyroid health is an issue, then avoid the recipes containing goitrogenic ingredients or make substitutions for other similar ingredients, such as swap kale for Swiss chard, peanut butter for almond butter, peaches for apricots, millet for oats or quinoa, etc. Raw eggs, which were used in preconception recipes, are no longer allowed in pregnancy smoothies; however, the use of dairy is okay. Moreover, the use of cacao is lessened in recipes in this chapter compared to the previous chapter due to stimulating effects. I have also provided recipes for both the first and third trimesters of pregnancy, as different nutrients are needed for those times. During the second trimester, the section on smoothies for whole pregnancy can be used.

Please note that recipes will vary in thickness and sweetness according to the choice of ingredients and this will vary further, particular with flavor, due to differences between seasons and produce quality. If you haven't read the introductory chapters before attempting my recipes, please go back and read them, particularly Chapter 1, "The Art and Science of Smoothies," which has detailed guidelines for my smoothie creations.

All recipes in this chapter yield 2 cups (500ml) that serve 1.

SMOOTHIES FOR WHOLE PREGNANCY

Certain nutrients are required throughout pregnancy to nourish the mother and ensure a good rate of growth for the child, including vitamins A, C, and B6, zinc, chromium, manganese, iodine, magnesium, selenium, protein, good fats, and probiotics.

The following smoothie recipes include ingredients that have these nutrients well covered—particularly if you add your probiotic to your smoothie.

Nectarine Nirvana

½ cup steamed or pureed sweet potato or pumpkin

¾ cup nectarine halves*

¼ inch slice fresh ginger

1 teaspoon vanilla extract or paste, or ½ vanilla bean

1 cup any milk

2 tablespoons hemp seeds

1–2 handfuls of spinach (optional)

*It's essential that nectarines are ripe, sweet, and juicy.

Citrus and Kiwi Cruiser

1 kiwi with skin, halved

1 packed cup mandarin orange segments

zest from ¼ lemon*

¼ avocado

6 ice cubes

sweeten to taste

handful of kale (optional)

*Use a vegetable peeler to remove zest.

Passion Fruit and Papaya Party

1 banana, frozen and sliced

¾ cup papaya

zest from ¼ lemon*

¾ cup coconut water

handful of parsley (optional)

pulp from 1 passion fruit**

*Use a vegetable peeler to remove zest.

**Blend all except passion fruit, which you stir through at the end by hand.

Orange and Mango Magician

1 cup mango flesh (about 1 mango)

¾ cup freshly squeezed orange juice

zest from ¼ lemon*

10 raw cashews

3 ice cubes

handful of fennel tops (optional)

*Use a vegetable peeler to remove zest.

Grape and Apple Glee

1 packed cup grapes

½ Granny Smith apple, quartered

1 tablespoon peanut butter

½ cup almond milk

¼ teaspoon ground Sri Lankan cinnamon

½ teaspoon ground turmeric

pinch of ground cardamom

4 ice cubes

1 bulb baby bok choy (optional), trimmed and well washed

Choccy Nutty Comfort

2 bananas, fresh or frozen and sliced

4 Brazil nuts*

1 heaping teaspoon raw cacao plus tiny pinch of salt

3 pitted prunes

1 cup any milk

1 serving plant-based protein powder

handful of Swiss chard (optional)

*Ideally, soak nuts overnight in water, then drain and rinse before use.

Creamy Protein Prize

2 tablespoons raw oats plus ½ cup water or milk, or ½ cup cooked oats, quinoa, or millet

1 banana, fresh or frozen and sliced

1 cup coconut water

3 tablespoons coconut cream

1 serving plant-based protein powder

1 teaspoon vanilla extract or paste, or ½ vanilla bean

Pleased as Peach

1 cup fresh* or steamed peach halves

½ cup fresh or frozen raspberries

¼ cup natural yogurt plus ½ cup milk, or ¾ cup milk kefir

1 teaspoon vanilla extract or paste, or ½ vanilla bean

sweeten to taste

handful of butter lettuce (optional)

*It's essential that the peaches are ripe, sweet, and juicy if used fresh.

THE FIRST TRIMESTER

The most important nutrients during the first trimester are B vitamins, namely folate, but also B2, B6, and B12. The following smoothies are designed to supply these essential nutrients. Unlike other recipes in this book, I haven't listed greens as optional as they are such a great source of folate and are very much recommended to use. Feel free to substitute the suggested leafy green, however; and for experienced green smoothie enthusiasts, feel free to use more than a handful of greens.

Yearning for Yogurt

2 bananas, fresh or frozen and sliced

¼ cup natural yogurt

½ cup any milk

1 teaspoon vanilla extract or paste, or ½ vanilla bean

1–2 handfuls of spinach

Christmas Pumpkin Pie

½ cup steamed or pureed sweet potato or pumpkin

1 cup freshly squeezed orange juice

10 raw cashews or 2 tablespoons hemp seeds

½ teaspoon ground Sri Lankan cinnamon

pinch of ground nutmeg

pinch of ground cloves

1 teaspoon vanilla extract or paste, or ½ vanilla bean

4 ice cubes

2 Chinese cabbage leaves, or 1 bulb baby bok choy, trimmed and well washed

Bonkers for Beets and Berries

¼ cup diced beet

1 cup any dark berry variety

¾ cup almond milk

6 walnut or pecan halves*

maple syrup to taste

3 ice cubes

*Ideally, soak overnight, drain, and rinse before blending.

Mango and Sunflower Surprise

1 banana

½ cup mango flesh

1 heaping tablespoon sunflower seeds*

¾ cup any milk

1 teaspoon vanilla extract or paste, or ½ vanilla bean

handful of beet greens

1–2 handfuls of butter lettuce

*Ideally, soak seeds overnight in water, then drain and rinse before use.

. . . .

3Ps: Pumpkin, Pear, and Peanuts

½ cup steamed or pureed sweet potato or pumpkin

1 pear, quartered

1 cup any milk

1 tablespoon peanut butter

handful of beet greens

sweeten to taste

1 heaping teaspoon raw cacao plus tiny punch of salt (optional)

. . . .

Precious Papaya

¾ cup papaya

1 banana, fresh or frozen and sliced

¼ cup coconut flesh and ¾ cup coconut water from a drinking coconut

squeeze of lemon juice

handful of romaine lettuce

. . . .

Creamy Banana Boost

2 bananas, fresh or frozen and sliced

¼ avocado

¾ cup any milk

1 teaspoon vanilla extract or paste, or ½ vanilla bean

handful of Swiss chard

. . . .

Super Seedy

1 cup freshly squeezed orange juice

½ cup diced raw or steamed carrot

1 tablespoon hemp seeds

1 tablespoon chia seeds

sweeten to taste

handful of parsley

. . . .

Mandarin and Melon Marvel

1 packed cup mandarin orange segments

1 cup cantaloupe

2 sprigs mint leaves

SMOOTHIES FOR NAUSEA

Around 70 percent of pregnant women experience nausea, with the majority just in the first trimester. If nausea is something you are dealing with, then these are the best smoothie recipes to try, due to the inclusion of magnesium and vitamin B6. Some are creamy to suit those who find fats helpful, and the others are cooling and fat free.

. . . .

Gratifying Grapes and Cucumber

2 cups frozen seedless grapes

1 large Persian cucumber, quartered

3–4 sprigs mint leaves

Honeydew Healer

1½ cups honeydew melon

¼ inch slice fresh ginger

4 ice cubes

1–2 handfuls of spinach (optional)

Watermelon Wow!

1½ cups watermelon

1½ cups any frozen berry

Quercetin Quencher

1 Granny Smith apple, cut into 8 pieces*

1 Persian cucumber, quartered

½ cup green seedless grapes

4 ice cubes

2–3 sprigs mint leaves (optional)

*If you dislike the mouthfeel of blended apples, you can try ¾ cup of apple juice instead.

4Cs: Carrot, Cucumber, Chia, and Chard

1 cup carrot juice

1 Persian cucumber, quartered

1 tablespoon chia seeds

3 ice cubes

handful of Swiss chard (optional)

Creamy Calm-a-rama

2 tablespoons raw oats plus ½ cup water or milk, or ½ cup cooked oats, quinoa, or millet

1 banana, fresh or frozen and sliced

10 raw cashews or 2 tablespoons hemps seeds

1 teaspoon vanilla extract or paste, or ½ vanilla bean

¼ teaspoon Sri Lankan cinnamon

1 cup any milk

3 medjool dates, pitted

handful of spinach (optional)

Fig and Ginger Freshener

1 packed cup fresh figs

¼ inch slice fresh ginger

¼ teaspoon ground Sri Lankan cinnamon

1 heaping tablespoon sunflower seeds, pumpkin seeds, or mixture*

1 cup any milk

3 ice cubes

maple syrup or stevia to taste

*Ideally, soak seeds overnight in water, then drain and rinse before use.

Spiced Surprise

½ cup steamed or pureed sweet potato or pumpkin

1 banana, fresh or frozen and sliced

¼ avocado

¼ inch slice fresh ginger

¼ teaspoon ground Sri Lankan cinnamon

1 teaspoon vanilla extract or paste, or ½ vanilla bean

1 cup any milk

handful of butter lettuce (optional)

Just Coconut and Berries

1½ cups frozen berries (any or mixed varieties)

½ cup coconut flesh and ¾ cup coconut water from a drinking coconut

Nausea Nurturer

1 tablespoon raw oats

1 banana, fresh or frozen and sliced

¼ cup full-fat natural yogurt

1 cup dairy milk

6 pitted prunes

¼ teaspoon ground Sri Lankan cinnamon

1 teaspoon vanilla extract or paste, or ½ vanilla bean

THE THIRD TRIMESTER

In the last trimester of pregnancy, nutrient demands are very high, as calcium, iron, DHA, vitamin E, and vitamin A in particular are transferred to the baby for storage and growth purposes. The following smoothies focus on ingredients rich in these nutrients, in addition to plenty of soluble fiber to combat constipation that frequently plagues late pregnancy. Please remember that omega-3 DHA will need to be sourced elsewhere in the diet with or without supplementation.

Party with Pears

2 fresh pears, quartered

2 fresh or dried figs*

1 tablespoon tahini

¼ teaspoon ground Sri Lankan cinnamon

thin slice fresh ginger

¾ cup any milk

handful of Swiss chard (optional)

*If using dried figs, soak overnight in ¼ cup of water and reduce milk to ½ cup.

Yogurt and Berry Bliss

1 cup frozen blueberries or raspberries

¼ cup natural yogurt plus ¾ cup non-dairy milk, or 1 cup milk kefir

1 heaping tablespoon sunflower seeds*

3 medjool dates, pitted

1–2 handfuls of spinach (optional)

*Ideally, soak seeds overnight in water, then drain and rinse before use.

Apple and Beet Boost

½ Granny Smith apple, quartered

1 cup green seedless grapes

¼ cup diced raw beet

½ cup almond milk

6 ice cubes

handful of kale (optional)

Citrus Soother

1 packed cup orange or mandarin orange segments

½ cup plum or nectarine halves*

1 teaspoon vanilla extract or paste, or ½ vanilla bean

¾ cup any milk

*It's essential that stone fruit is ripe, sweet, and juicy.

Kiwi Kooler

1 Persian cucumber, quartered

2 kiwi with skin, halved

¾ cup coconut water

3 ice cubes

3 sprigs mint leaves

Strawberry and Papaya Pleasure

1½ cups/1 punnet strawberries with hulls

¾ cup papaya

¼ avocado

squeeze of lemon or lime juice

Apricot and Mango Marvel

½ cup apricot halves, fresh or steamed

½ cup mango flesh

1 passion fruit*

1 tablespoon chia seeds

4 Brazil nuts**

½ teaspoon ground turmeric

1 cup any milk

*Blend all ingredients except passion fruit, which you stir through at the end by hand.

**Ideally, soak nuts overnight, discard water, and rinse well.

Moving and Grooving

2 tablespoons raw rolled oats, 4 prunes and 2 dried apricots soaked in 1¼ cups milk* overnight in the fridge

1 banana, fresh or frozen and sliced

2 tablespoons hemp seeds

¼ teaspoon ground Sri Lankan cinnamon

1 teaspoon vanilla extract or paste, or ½ vanilla bean

*Any milk except coconut milk.

CARDIOVASCULAR-FRIENDLY SMOOTHIES

The health of the cardiovascular system is very important while pregnant, with 50 percent greater blood volume produced and organs working much harder, so it's little wonder tiredness and swelling is very common. The key smoothie-friendly nutrients to maintain healthy blood volume, manage blood pressure, and keep homocysteine down include B2, B6, folate, choline, magnesium, potassium, zinc, and iron.

Pink Porridge

½ cup cold porridge

¼ cup diced raw beet

1 cup strawberries with hulls

3 tablespoons coconut cream

½ cup coconut water

handful of beet leaves (optional)

Papaya and Lime Lifter

1 banana, fresh or frozen and sliced

¾ cup papaya

zest from ¼ lime*

¾ cup coconut milk

*Use a vegetable peeler to remove zest.

Peanut and Turmeric Temptation

½ cup steamed or pureed sweet potato or pumpkin

1 banana, fresh or frozen and sliced

1 tablespoon peanut butter

4 prunes, pitted, or 2 medjool dates, pitted

½ teaspoon ground turmeric

1 cup almond milk

handful of butter lettuce (optional)

Lemon and Raspberry Revelation

2 tablespoons raw oats plus ½ cup water or milk, or ½ cup cooked oats, quinoa, or millet

¾ cup frozen raspberries

zest from ½ lemon*

1 teaspoon vanilla extract or paste, or ½ vanilla bean

¼ cup natural yogurt plus ¾ cup milk, or 1 cup milk kefir

honey or maple syrup to taste

1 bulb baby bok choy (optional), trimmed and well washed

*Use a vegetable peeler to remove zest.

Goji Gold

2 bananas, fresh or frozen and sliced

½ cup coconut milk

2 tablespoons goji berries soaked in ¼ cup water (keep water)

1 tablespoon chia seeds

handful of romaine lettuce (optional)

Ginger and Pumpkin Party

2 dried figs with stem tips removed, soaked in 1 cup any milk overnight in the fridge

½ cup steamed or pureed sweet potato or pumpkin

1 banana, fresh or frozen and sliced

¼ inch slice fresh ginger

. . . .

Chocolate Mint Fix

1 large banana, frozen and sliced

6 prunes, pitted, or 3 medjool dates, pitted

1 heaping teaspoon raw cacao plus tiny pinch of salt

10 raw cashews

1 cup any milk or water

3–4 sprigs mint leaves

. . . .

Spicy Carrot Creation

2 tablespoons raw oats, plus 3 tablespoons raisins soaked in 1 cup any milk overnight in the fridge

½ cup carrot juice

¼ teaspoon ground Sri Lankan cinnamon

pinch of ground nutmeg

1 teaspoon vanilla extract or paste, or ½ vanilla bean

1 tablespoon hulled tahini or 2 tablespoons hemp seeds

handful of kale (optional)

. . . .

Macadamia and Mandarin Monster

½ cup steamed or pureed sweet potato or pumpkin

1 cup mandarin orange segments

5 raw macadamias

¾ cup any milk (except coconut)

1 teaspoon vanilla extract or paste, or ½ vanilla bean

3 ice cubes

1–2 handfuls of spinach (optional)

SKIN-SAVING SMOOTHIES

If you have not been blessed with clear, bright skin during pregnancy or you are at risk of stretch marks, try these smoothie recipes full of skin supportive nutrients like vitamins A, C, and E, biotin, silica, and zinc.

. . . .

Beaming with Beets

½ cup diced raw beet

1 packed cup seedless grapes

¾ cup almond milk

4 ice cubes

4 walnut or pecan halves*

1 tablespoon chia seeds

*Ideally, soak overnight, drain, and rinse before blending.

. . . .

Bust Out with Bananas

2 bananas, frozen and sliced

¼ cup natural yogurt plus ½ cup milk, or ¾ cup milk kefir

1 teaspoon vanilla extract or paste, or ½ vanilla bean

1–2 Chinese cabbage leaves (optional)

Papaya Coconut Connection

¾ cup papaya

1 large banana, fresh or frozen and sliced

squeeze of lemon or lime juice

¾ cup water or coconut water

3 tablespoons coconut cream

handful of Swiss chard (optional)

Nut and Seed Sensation

½ cup steamed or pureed sweet potato or pumpkin

1 pear, quartered (must be soft and juicy)

1 tablespoon peanut butter

2 teaspoons chia seeds

½ teaspoon ground turmeric

1 cup almond milk

1 bulb baby bok choy, trimmed and well washed

Glow with Mango

1 banana, fresh or frozen and sliced

½ cup mango flesh

1 heaping tablespoon sunflower seeds

1 cup any milk

1 teaspoon vanilla extract or paste, or ½ vanilla bean

1–2 handfuls of spinach (optional)

*Ideally, soak seeds overnight in water, then drain and rinse before use.

. . . .

Mandarin Mayhem

1 packed cup mandarin orange segments

1 packed cup cantaloupe

handful of romaine lettuce (optional)

. . . .

Carrot and Citrus Sizzle

½ cup steamed carrot*

1½ cups freshly squeezed orange juice

2 tablespoons hemp seeds

1 teaspoon vanilla extract or paste, or ½ vanilla bean

¼ teaspoon ground Sri Lankan cinnamon

pinch of ground cloves

sweeten to taste (shouldn't be needed if you have really good oranges)

handful of parsley (optional)

*Frozen cubes of cooked carrot will work well in this recipe.

. . . .

Banana Calmer

2 bananas, frozen and sliced

¼ avocado

¾ cup any milk

1 teaspoon vanilla extract or paste, or ½ vanilla bean

SMOOTHIES FOR CRAMPS

The following recipes are designed to help manage the tendency in later pregnancy to experience leg muscle cramps, and are replete in the key nutrients required: potassium, magnesium, and calcium.

. . . .

Muscle Meditation

2 bananas, fresh or frozen and sliced

4 Brazil nuts*

1 heaping teaspoon raw cacao plus tiny pinch of salt

¼ cup young coconut flesh or 3 tablespoons coconut cream

¾ cup coconut water

handful of Swiss chard

*Ideally, soak nuts overnight, discard water, and rinse well.

. . . .

Beet My Berries

1 cup fresh blackberries

¼ cup diced raw beet

¾ cup any milk

1 tablespoon hulled tahini

1 tablespoon chia seeds

3 medjool dates, pitted

3 ice cubes

handful of beet leaves (optional)

Berry Creamy

1 cup any frozen berry or mixed frozen berries

1 large pear, quartered

¼ cup natural yogurt plus ½ cup milk, or ¾ cup milk kefir

sweeten to taste

Sweet Potato Pleasure

½ cup steamed or pureed sweet potato or pumpkin

1 banana, fresh or frozen and sliced

¼ avocado

1 cup coconut water

1 teaspoon vanilla extract or paste, or ½ vanilla bean

handful of butter lettuce

Peach and Tahini Tantalizer

1 cup fresh or steamed peach halves*

1 banana, fresh or frozen and sliced

1 tablespoon hulled tahini

¾ cup any milk (except coconut)

1 teaspoon vanilla extract or paste, or ½ vanilla bean

thin slice fresh ginger (optional)

*It's essential that peaches are ripe, sweet, and juicy if used fresh.

Vanilla Yogurt Euphoria

2 bananas, fresh or frozen and sliced

¼ cup natural yogurt plus ½ cup milk, or ¾ cup milk kefir

1 teaspoon vanilla extract or paste, or ½ vanilla bean

sweeten to taste

1–2 handfuls of spinach

Raspberry Relaxer

1 cup frozen raspberries

1 banana or pear, quartered

2 tablespoons hemp seeds

¾ cup coconut water

2–3 sprigs mint leaves

Choc-Banana Chill-Out

2 tablespoons raw oats plus ½ cup water or milk, or ½ cup cooked oats, quinoa, or millet

1 banana, fresh or frozen and sliced

1 cup any milk

1 heaped teaspoon raw cacao plus tiny pinch of salt

1 tablespoon any nut butter

3 medjool dates, pitted

pinch of ground nutmeg

handful of kale or other brassica

The Avocado Advantage

1 banana, fresh or frozen and sliced

½ avocado

1 cup coconut water

1 teaspoon vanilla extract or paste, or ½ vanilla bean

handful of Swiss chard

MOOD-BOOSTING SMOOTHIES

Pregnancy can be an emotional time and if struggling with feeling low, it's important to seek help, in addition to including mood-boosting nutrients such as vitamin B6, vitamin C, folate, zinc, tyrosine, tryptophan, protein, and good fats, which are all included in the following smoothie recipes.

Banana and Protein Punch

1 banana, fresh or frozen and sliced

¼ avocado

1 serving plant-based protein powder

1 cup coconut water

1 teaspoon vanilla extract or paste, or ½ vanilla bean

Sunny Strawberries and Cream

2 tablespoons raw rolled oats plus ½ cup milk, or ½ cup porridge

1½ cups/1 punnet strawberries with hulls

¼ cup full-fat natural yogurt plus ¼ cup any milk, or ½ cup milk kefir

3 medjool dates, pitted

pulp of 1 passion fruit*

*Blend all except passion fruit, which you stir through at the end by hand.

Peaceful Papaya

1 packed cup papaya

¼ cup coconut flesh and ¾ cup coconut water from a drinking coconut

¼ inch slice fresh ginger

1 bulb baby bok choy (optional), trimmed and well washed

Cheerful Cherries

1 banana, fresh or frozen and sliced

1 cup pitted cherries

¾ cup any milk or water

10 raw cashews

1–2 handfuls of spinach (optional)

Spicy Sweet Potato

½ cup steamed or pureed sweet potato or pumpkin

¾ cup mango flesh

2 tablespoons hemp seeds

¼ teaspoon ground Sri Lankan cinnamon

pinch of ground nutmeg

pinch of ground cloves

1 cup any milk

. . . .

Fig and Ginger Fun

1 banana, frozen and sliced

3 fresh figs, stem tips removed

1 serving plant-based protein powder

¼ teaspoon ground Sri Lankan cinnamon

thin slice fresh ginger*

1 cup almond milk

handful of butter lettuce (optional)

. . . .

Fun with Fennel

1½ cups beet and fennel juice

1–2 handfuls of fennel tops

8 raw macadamias

1 tablespoon chia seeds

4 ice cubes

. . . .

Banana Choc Content

2 bananas, fresh or frozen and sliced

1 heaping teaspoon raw cacao plus tiny pinch of salt

1 tablespoon pumpkin seeds*

1 tablespoon hulled tahini

¾ cup coconut water

2 medjool dates, pitted

2–3 sprigs mint leaves (optional)

*Ideally, soak seeds overnight in water, then drain and rinse before use.

. . . .

Choc Full of Muesli

½ cup raw muesli*

1 banana

1 cup non-dairy milk

1 heaping teaspoon raw cacao plus tiny pinch of salt

1 egg (optional)

*If time permits, soak the muesli in the milk in the fridge overnight, which will result in a creamier smoothie made the next day.

CHAPTER 5

After the Baby Is Born

Congratulations! Your baby has arrived (or babies if you had multiples)! The postnatal period has two important themes: One is your recovery post-birth, be it natural, assisted vaginal, or via caesarean section; and then there is breastfeeding. This chapter is written with the assumption that breastfeeding is occurring. This is because nutritional and calorie requirements are different for a mother who isn't breastfeeding, whose diet can be considered "normal," albeit ideally well balanced and healthy. If you are not breastfeeding, the smoothie recipes suggested will still be beneficial as they are all designed to be highly nourishing, which is important for all new mothers.

During preconception there is the forward planning to become pregnant, then once that is achieved, the focus is on what's happening now and what's happening next with respect to the baby's development. Then of course, there is a huge focus on the birth itself: Birth plans are written (or not), choices are made for hospital or home births, water births, calm births, hypnobirths, and caesarean births. There are decisions regarding delayed or immediate cord clamping, post-birth vaccinations, and use of drugs. Do you do perineal massage? Who will be there at the birth? What's your plan once labor starts? What's in your hospital bag? Have you packed a hospital bag? Will you use a gym ball, or a TENS (transcutaneous electrical nerve stimulation) machine? The list goes on and on.

Between all this birth planning and getting "stuff"—the crib, bassinet, bouncy chair, changeable diapers, car seat, stroller, baby carrier, clothing, spew cloths, swaddle cloths, blankets, etc.—it's little wonder that the "doing" part of looking after a baby is not so well prepared for, such as managing birth recovery and developing the skill of breastfeeding.

Then there's the emotional roller coaster postnatally. You think you are emotional while pregnant, well for many that's nothing compared to after the baby is born! All my friends warned me about uncontrollable crying on day 3 or 4 post-birth and they weren't kidding: I could look at the wall and cry. Then being discharged from the hospital that same day didn't help matters! It got easier after that but whether I was tired, scared, or having a moment of joy, the tears would come. I am pretty certain I cried most days for the first 6 weeks—granted I had a baby in the hospital, but I know plenty of new mothers with "normal" births that were much the same as a result of sleep deprivation, nipple pain, birth-related pain, and plunging hormone levels.

So where do smoothies fit in during the postnatal period? Given smoothies are quick to prepare and you can pack a lot into them, they tick two important boxes: You will be short on time and your nutritional and caloric needs will be increased. Smoothies are also a great way to consume "lactogenic" foods to help maintain or increase breast milk supply.

Since having my son, I have found smoothies to be a lifesaver.
They have meant that, without too much time and effort on
my behalf, I am able to have a nutrition-packed breakfast
that can keep me going until lunchtime without snacking.
This is great because I find it hard to get the time to prepare
snacks, healthy or otherwise, and I know that if I didn't have
the smoothie I would resort to bought snacks, which would
not allow me to lose and keep off the weight I gained during
my pregnancy. It's also great to know that when I'm getting
great nutrition, so is bubs through my breast milk. —Sarah

Your Hospital Stay

Unless you had a homebirth, you will have to face the notoriously
terrible hospital food. It's bland, it has tiny portions, and it is
far from healthy. Visitors such as family and close friends will
ask what they can do to help, so ask them to bring you food and
drinks! You will need high-energy, protein-, and fat-based snacks
such as bliss balls made of nuts, dates, and coconut. You will
need hydrating liquids, such as coconut water and good-quality
mineral or filtered water, and you will need greens. Greens are
alkaline, mineral-rich, detoxifying (important to help get rid of any
drugs you may have ended up having), and very healing. If you
can get someone to bring you a green smoothie each day, that's
a great start. You can usually pick lunches and dinners off the
hospital menu that are protein- and vegetable-based and avoid the
processed carbohydrates. However, breakfast options are usually
very limited and very ordinary, so this is your best time to drink
that smoothie. Even if it's brought in the night before, a smoothie
can go in the fridge on the ward in a glass jar or a stainless-steel
drink bottle and will be fine the next morning—give it a shake and

ideally let it warm up to room temperature. Short of that, take some powdered greens with you to mix up with water or juice a couple of times a day. My preferred brand is Miessence Deep Green Alkalising Superfood, which is organic and uses grass juice powder not grass powder. Big tubs of green powders are not really value for money as they are not concentrated, often contain non-nutritive fillers, and as a grass powder, they have indigestible components like cellulose.

Post-Birth Swelling

For approximately a week post-birth you will have a lot of lower limb swelling. During pregnancy your body produces 50 percent more blood, and after the baby is born this is no longer needed; so as the body adjusts, fluid will collect in your extremities but won't tend to settle in the morning and increase at night like during pregnancy—it will be consistent and gradually reduce. Keep up plenty of fluids, move around as tolerated, and consume celery. Celery is a diuretic (removes fluids via the urine) and though diuretics are thought to dry up breast milk, the fluid retention post-birth is thought to delay milk production; hence, the use of celery will indirectly act as a galactagogue (stimulating breast milk production) in this situation. In a smoothie, celery ribs and/ or leaves can be used though they are quite fibrous and strong in flavor. Celery juice may also be used as part of the liquid base.

Hair Loss

From around 6 weeks post-birth most women experience significant hair loss and it can go on and on for many months. Mine stopped around 5 months postpartum, but I have heard of some women reporting hair loss after 1 year. This phenomenon has nothing to do with nutrition—it's hormonal. When pregnant, high estrogen levels causes the usual hair loss to slow down, which is normally about 100 hairs a day. Once estrogen takes a dive after birth, the falling-out process starts up again and makes up for lost time! This is of course why your hair gets thicker (everywhere!) during pregnancy too.

Hair loss can also be a symptom of thyroid disorders, which can also play up during and after pregnancy, so if you have a known thyroid condition it's best to get tested in case medication requires adjusting. Hair loss can also be a symptom of iron deficiency. In the absence of anemia or a thyroid problem, the hair loss can still be quite alarming. I remember it coming out in clumps after the shower and it was always clogging up the vacuum cleaner! But rest assured, it will stop eventually, though there is not much you can do about it in the meantime.

If your hair loss relates to a thyroid issue or iron deficiency, thyroid-friendly smoothies and iron-rich smoothies are a great way to consume the nutrients you require. As previously discussed, vitamins A, B12, C, D, and E, the amino acid tyrosine, the minerals selenium, iodine, magnesium and zinc, and coconut oil are all important nutrients for optimal thyroid function.

Smoothie- and postnatal-friendly iron sources: eggs, leafy greens (especially spinach, Swiss chard, and parsley), dried apricots, raisins, prunes, beets, cacao, blackstrap molasses, pumpkin seeds, oats, chia, and quinoa

Appetite

Post-birth you will likely be crazy hungry! This is something no one told me, yet most breastfeeding mothers say they were, too.

Depending on your source, you will need 300 to 600 more calories over the first 3 months while breastfeeding. What I did was to start my day with a big green smoothie (even though I wasn't living at home while my baby was in the hospital, I had a blender with me and still made smoothies), and had a good-sized lunch and dinner based on vegetables and protein. In between meals I snacked on lactation cookies (more on that later). I did go through a stage of eating more chocolate than the odd piece, so I had to nip that one in the bud! The desire for sugar can be quite intense especially if not drinking tea or coffee, as tiredness, stress, and not eating often enough can affect blood sugar. Drinking tea or coffee as an energy boost isn't recommended either, as caffeine will enter your breast milk and may make the baby cranky, or keep them awake when you want them to sleep! Chocolate frequently has the same effect.

> After having a pregnancy affected by nausea at the start
> and heartburn at the end, I had seriously limited the foods
> I could eat, including the content of my smoothies, and my
> portions had drastically reduced compared to normal. It was
> a relief to be able to eat and drink normally again, but the
> hunger I had far surpassed anything I had ever experienced
> before! This might explain why I had a flatter stomach 3
> to 4 weeks post-birth than at 3 to 4 months! —Kate

Recovery

Basic vaginal recovery from stretching and mild tearing usually takes 2 to 4 weeks, with more serious trauma taking much longer, and possibly leaving scaring for life. Caesarean sections involve cutting through and sewing up seven layers, and generally takes 6 weeks to recover, with most women feeling pretty good after 2 to 4 weeks also.

Protein is important for growth and repair, in particular repair from traumatic vaginal births or caesarean sections. Protein will help your scars heal, and because protein spends longer in the stomach than carbohydrates, it slows down carbohydrate digestion, which is good for steady blood sugar. Protein is also more satiating than carbohydrate, so you are less likely to overeat with protein at each meal. In a smoothie, protein can be via the addition of greens (but needs to be a couple of good handfuls, not just a little handful), whole nuts and seeds or nut and seed milks, raw eggs, and/or protein powders. As discussed in Chapter 4, "Knocked Up," protein requirements while pregnant and lactating are around 1g per kg of body weight (0.5g per pound) per day.

Fats and oils, as we know, are needed from preconception to breastfeeding, with smoothie-friendly "good fats" being those rich in omega-3 ALA (chia, flax, and hemp), omega-6 GLA (hemp), and monounsaturated fats (macadamia, avocado, and almond). Anti–inflammatory GLA is in breast milk and is dependent upon the mother's diet, as is omega-3 DHA, which will need to come primarily from other parts of the diet and supplementing (discussed in more detail later in this chapter).

Stress

Stress is something that can be a significant issue in the postpartum period. Juggling many tasks and sleep deprivation can take its toll, especially if you have an unsettled baby. DHA consumption is important as "brain food" (see Chapter 2, "Fabulous Fats"); hence it's essential to eat DHA-rich foods *and* supplement at least 200mg to 300mg per day, to ensure you are getting enough to reduce the risk of postnatal depression, and so it gets into your breast milk for your baby too.

When stress levels are consistently high, you will risk adrenal fatigue. Your adrenal glands sit on your kidneys and produce hormones such as adrenalin and noradrenaline, which control the "fight or flight" response. The release of these hormones is not designed to be constant and high, but when they are, the adrenal glands run out of steam and start failing to produce enough when you do need it. Symptoms can include feeling weak, tiredness not relieved by sleep, dizziness when rising, cravings for salty foods, depression, and gastrointestinal upset.

Managing the stress of motherhood can be easier said than done, but delegating duties and asking for help is key. Nutritionally, you can nourish your adrenals by avoiding caffeine, alcohol, sugar, and excessive grain-based carbohydrates. Furthermore, you can add adrenal-supportive nutrients to your smoothies.

Smoothie-friendly and postpartum stress-busting sources: For DHA, raw eggs from chickens raised on pasture; coconut oil for its beneficial saturated fats; pumpkin and sunflower seeds for zinc; dairy milk, yogurt, seeds, bananas, and avocados for tyrosine; cashews, chia seeds, and leafy greens for magnesium; fruits for vitamin C; and leafy greens, eggs, and bananas for B vitamins. Licorice root is also beneficial for the adrenals and can be made up as a tea and used as a smoothie liquid base. If not eating or minimally consuming animal products or you have known low B12, then supplementing B12 is essential—see Chapter 3, "Making Babies," for more on absorption issues of B12.

Breastfeeding

Breastfeeding is physically, emotionally, and hormonally charged! For some it comes easily with no issues: baby latches and is settled during and after feeds. For others it is hard work. Furthermore, breastfeeding versus formula feeding is fraught with emotion and politics, with those who chest beat (pardon the pun) the "breast is best" message to those who embrace formula feeding very happily. The fact is, breast milk is best, but it's not always possible. Only a small percentage of women truly can't breastfeed or find it very difficult, due to inadequate glandular breast tissue, retained placenta, or uncontrolled medical conditions such as thyroid disorders, PCOS, or diabetes—which affect the balance of hormones required to breastfeed. Otherwise it's usually due to severe latching difficulties or untreated significant tongue/lip tie. Some women choose not to breastfeed at all or give up on breastfeeding for various reasons, such as unbearable nipple trauma, baby losing weight, milk drying up early, not enjoying it, peer pressure to stop, having a very unsettled baby, returning to work, etc.

Compared to formula feeding, breastfeeding reduces the risk of obesity, celiac disease, diabetes, cardiovascular disease, cancer, respiratory and ear infections, and meningitis. Plus, it reduces the risk of stress disorders and osteoporosis in the mother. Breast milk is antibacterial, antiviral, anti-inflammatory, boosts the effect of vaccinations, and is allergy protective when provided in combination with solid foods for baby, particularly gluten and the proteins in wheat, barley, oats, and rye.

Formula is not evil and it does nourish an infant. If it didn't provide nourishment, it would not be for sale. However, it is significantly different from human breast milk: There are no enzymes or immune protective properties in formula; there is no genetic match; and the milk is the same all the time—versus breast milk, which is watery at first and gets fattier over a feed, over the day, and in the second year of lactation. The lower-fat portion of the milk is also called the foremilk, which exits the breast first, versus the higher-fat hind milk that is the latter part of

Incidence of Breastfeeding

The World Health Organization (WHO) "recommends mothers worldwide to exclusively breastfeed infants for the child's first 6 months to achieve optimal growth, development, and health. Thereafter, they should be given nutritious complementary foods and continue breastfeeding up to the age of 2 years or beyond" (www.who.int/en). This is supported by the United Nations Children's Fund (UNICEF), the Department of Health in the United Kingdom, the American Academy of Pediatrics (AAP), and the NHMRC in Australia. Given this worldwide recommendation, it is surprising to see what actually is occurring:

- Conducted in 2010–11, the Australian National Infant Feeding Survey reported breastfeeding was initiated in 96 percent of infants. Only 39 percent were exclusively breastfed by 3 months, and 15 percent by 6 months.

- In the United States, the Centers for Disease Control and Prevention (CDC) breastfeeding report card states that the breastfeeding initiation rate is 76.9 percent. Exclusive breastfeeding at 3 months was 36 percent and at 6 months was 16 percent.

- In the UK, the National Health Service (NHS) infant feeding survey of 2010 reported 81 percent breastfeeding initiation. At 3 months, 17 percent were exclusively breastfeeding, and at 6 months, only 1 percent.

- A common reason for ceasing or reducing breastfeeding is reporting a drop in supply. As will be discussed later in this chapter, these drops in supply are frequently perceptions only and understanding this concept could mean improvement in breastfeeding rates.

the feed. Formula frequently has genetically modified ingredients and has poor bioavailability of nutrients like calcium, iron, and zinc. Mother's milk has the flavors and aromas of the mother's diet, which is believed to positively influence dietary preferences of the child once on solids. Non-human fats are not protective to the nervous system and formula-fed infants are prone to being fatter.

In Australia there are calls to put warning labels on formula cans and packaging, namely highlighting links to obesity, and the risk that supplementing breastfeeding with formula can deplete breast milk supply.

STAGES OF LACTATION

Follow any number of online parenting forums and you will note a common topic of needing to increase milk supply, with some good advice given and lots of misinformed advice, too. If starting and continuing to breastfeed is a priority for you, then understanding how milk production works is essential, including how nutrition can be of influence for quality and quantity, and how smoothies can play an important and convenient role.

The first stage of lactation is called mammogenesis. This stage actually begins during puberty when breasts begin to grow with exposure to estrogen. Subsequent high levels of estrogen during pregnancy stimulate an increase in prolactin levels, which prepare the breast for the potential to feed a baby, via the division and proliferation of glandular tissue cells. This stage is complete during the third trimester of pregnancy.

The second stage is called lactogenesis I, which heralds the beginnings of colostrum production around 10 to 12 weeks gestation. Colostrum is thick, yellow, and full of protective antibodies. The breast is capable of producing colostrum from around the fourth month of pregnancy. Colostrum helps the baby pass "meconium," the first sticky, thick black poo. It also offers protection to the lining of the gut and helps establish bifidus, the friendly bacteria essential to an infant's gut. Colostrum is high in protein, carotenoids, sodium, chloride, potassium, zinc, and vitamins A and E. It is lower in lactose, fat, and water-soluble vitamins compared to mature breast milk.

The third stage is lactogenesis II, the establishment of milk supply 2 to 4 days post-birth and specifically following the delivery of the placenta due to the sudden withdrawal of hormones, particularly progesterone, which when high during pregnancy opposes prolactin, the hormone responsible for milk production. This third stage occurs independently of a baby suckling and is referred to as "the milk coming in."

The fourth stage, called lactogenesis III, is the maturation of milk production and supply, also known previously as galactopoiesis, and is dependent on the baby feeding (or via expressing with a pump or manually). This stage develops over the first 2 weeks post-birth, and the synthesis of milk will increase according to supply and demand, or the frequency *and* extent that milk is drained from the breasts. There is a substance in breast milk called feedback inhibitor of lactation (FIL) that is higher in a full breast. A full breast signals a slowing of milk production, versus an emptied breast signaling milk production to speed up. This is why it's important to feed (or pump) frequently in the early weeks, i.e., 8 to 12 times daily, and aim to drain at least one breast per feed to avoid raised FIL levels.

THE ROLES OF LACTATION HORMONES

The pituitary gland in the brain is responsible for the synthesis of prolactin, the hormone that facilitates milk production. The pituitary also releases oxytocin, which is a hormone that is responsible for the "let down" or "milk ejection reflex." This reflex results in contraction of smooth muscle in the breasts to squeeze the milk into ducts toward the nipple. Let down occurs namely from direct nipple stimulation/sucking, but can occur without, and both breasts will let down together. Receptors in and around the nipple send signals to the hypothalamus in the brain, and the hypothalamus controls the pituitary gland. Nipple suckling triggers the process that leads to the release of oxytocin from the pituitary to facilitate let down, while the same suckling triggers a rise in prolactin to help fill the breast for the next feed. Prolactin peaks during REM sleep and early in the morning, which is why sleep (as opposes to just rest) helps milk production. Oxytocin, on the other hand, can be affected by stress as it requires a relaxed state to facilitate let down, and in turn oxytocin is relaxing and helps reduce stress, so it can be a bit of a catch-22. Bottom line is your stress levels would need to be very high, in combination with less frequent nursing, to result in a significant loss of milk supply. Something as simple as taking a few deep breaths as you start to breastfeed can aid let down, but in more serious cases, relaxation techniques of meditation can be very useful. Fennel (in tea or tincture form) may also aid let down, as can the use of a rescue remedy before a feed.

Oxytocin is also responsible for contraction of the uterus in labor for giving birth, and while breastfeeding to help the uterus shrink back to normal. Oxytocin is considered to be a "mothering" or "bonding" hormone. Its influence is calming. It reduces blood pressure, cortisol levels, anxiety, and aggressive tendencies— hence, it's a very important hormone to help cope with the demands of being a new parent. But it's not just for mothers: Studies have shown that fathers' levels of oxytocin can be as high as mothers', but it is released via stimulatory and exploratory play, such as playing airplanes and stimulating laughter together. In contrast, a mother's oxytocin release is related to breastfeeding and affection, such as cuddles, light tickles, and gazing into each other's eyes. Fathers are prone to postnatal depression, too, so active playtime with their baby is very important for their mental health and bonding.

BREAST MILK QUALITY

The single most important factor when it comes to breast milk production is supply and demand—not nutrition, water consumption, or even rest. Advice to drink plenty of fluids to maintain milk supply is erroneous, and drinking milk certainly does not make milk! Lactation resources consistently state to drink to thirst, and in fact too much fluid is linked to reduced milk production. If not enough water is being consumed, the mother will end up dehydrated but her volume of milk will be the same. This is not ideal, of course, for the mother's health, but the baby will be fine.

With regard to hydration and nutrition, the body will always prioritize the quality of milk, and only in cases of severe dehydration or malnutrition will milk quality be significantly affected. Malnourished mothers from poor socioeconomic situations, some teen mothers (who are still developing and have higher nutritional needs yet often eat poorly), or those with anorexia/bulimia or drug users will have less of the water-soluble vitamins (Bs and C), vitamin D, lactose, and fat.

The levels of protein, total fats, antibodies, iron, chromium, calcium, phosphates, magnesium, potassium sodium, chloride, sulfates, and citrates in breast milk are not affected by the mother's diet while breastfeeding. Slightly dependent on the mother's diet are the fat-soluble vitamins A, E, and K, chromium, iodine, manganese, selenium, and zinc.

What is dependent on the mother's diet while breastfeeding is fatty acid consumption, namely omega-3 DHA, vitamins D and C, and the B vitamins, especially B12. In smoothies, DHA, vitamin D, and B12 can come from raw grass-fed chicken eggs, but these three nutrients often require supplementation as previously discussed. Vitamin C is abundant in fruits and some leafy greens. Leafy greens will also supply minerals and variable amounts of B vitamins. Dairy products are not naturally a good source of vitamin D, but many commercial types of milk will be fortified. Dairy, however, is the most common allergen to infants and frequently a source of sensitivity in breast milk, so for many it needs to be avoided. Vitamin D deficiency in an infant can be corrected through breast milk if the mother takes a high dose (the prescription of which should be through an appropriate health professional).

IMMUNE-BOOSTING NUTRIENTS

Ingredients of mother's milk that are dependent on the mother's diet are ones that are particularly important for immunity, namely vitamins A, Bs, C, D, and E, plus the minerals iodine, manganese, selenium, and zinc. It's imperative that the diet of a breastfeeding mother is replete with these nutrients to ensure she remains healthy, as well as passing on necessary nutrients to her baby. Plant foods supply all of these requirements with the richest smoothie-friendly sources for the postpartum period listed below:

Smoothie-friendly vitamin A sources: eggs, carrots, pumpkin, sweet potato, spinach, kale, cantaloupe, mango, papaya, pineapples, passion fruit, apricots, peaches, nectarines, and kiwi

Smoothie-friendly vitamin C sources: brassicas (such as kale and collards), parsley, papaya, avocado, passion fruit, beets, pomegranates, strawberries, mangoes, bananas, kiwi, citrus, and melons

Smoothie-friendly vitamin D sources: eggs (and sunshine!)

Smoothie-friendly vitamin E sources: leafy greens (especially chard and spinach), avocado, sunflower seeds, almonds, peanuts, mint, papaya, kiwi, nectarines, and raspberries

Smoothie-friendly manganese sources: cinnamon, pineapple, passion fruit, strawberries, turmeric, oats, sweet potato, kiwi, beets, and leafy greens (especially spinach and brassicas)

Smoothie-friendly zinc sources: blackstrap molasses, cacao, chia, coconut, cashews, Swiss chard, spinach, parsley, eggs, macadamias, maple syrup, oats, pecans, peanuts, hemp seeds, pumpkin seeds, tahini, figs, ginger root, almonds, and sunflower seeds

Smoothie-friendly selenium sources: Brazil nuts, sunflower seeds, eggs, cashews, macadamias, and oats

Note: Cod liver oil is an excellent natural source of both vitamins A and D, and though not smoothie-friendly, it makes a good food-based supplement (versus synthetically made in a lab).

Ensuring your postpartum diet is rich in these nutrients is essential for the immunity of your baby via your milk, and also for you, as they will reduce the risk of infections such as colds, flus, and tummy bugs. I strongly believe that the reason my daughter had not a single infection associated with her condition while in the hospital or afterward, and was discharged after 8 weeks and not the estimated 6 months, was due to breastfeeding exclusively and ensuring my diet was replete with these particular nutrients.

PROBIOTICS

Probiotics taken by a mother also influences the amount of probiotics in breast milk. These "friendly bacteria" are essential for immunity, and countless numbers exist in the gut. If you or your baby has been on antibiotics, they are paramount to take. There are probiotics that are based on bifidus that can be given to a young baby. Bifidus is the predominant bacteria in a baby's gut in the first 6 months, which assists with the digestion of breast milk. After this a baby's gut evolves to include less bifidus and more other species, such as lactobacillus, and functions more like an adult gut. Probiotics for mothers can be consumed in the form of capsules or powders, or in the form of fermented foods and drinks such as kefir, which can, like capsules or powders, be easily added to smoothie recipes. I take probiotics twice daily and the morning dose always goes in my smoothie.

REDUCTION IN MILK SUPPLY AND FALSE PERCEPTIONS

When it comes to longevity with breastfeeding, it's imperative to understand the difference between a genuine reduction in milk supply versus a perceived one. If it's only perceived then subsequent actions can be detrimental to supply, such as the addition of a supplementary feed (formula or from stored expressed milk). Just a single bottle can have a negative affect due to the reduction of breast stimulation from suckling. The classic example is using a supplementary feed in the late evening because your supply is lower at that time of day. One less feed is one less opportunity for prolactin to be released, and if this is combined with your baby sleeping through the night, you may go 10 to 12 hours without nursing, which may have further detrimental effects. The saving grace in this situation can be that prolactin is highest overnight and released when in REM sleep; however, such long periods of no nursing, especially before solids are well established, risk supply, as well as the development of blocked ducts or mastitis. Returning to work, even part time, can also affect milk supply for the same reasons, as it can be difficult to express at the times you usually nurse and the usual frequency of nursing.

Perceived self-weaning: It should be noted, that despite reports of ceasing breastfeeding due to baby "self-weaning," this phenomenon is truly rare before 1 year, when milk is still the predominant source of nutrition. What can happen is misinterpretation of a nursing strike, when the baby suddenly stops feeding. This can happen for many reasons, including the baby being unwell or in pain. There are numerous strategies described to combat the different reasons, and an excellent source of information about this can be found at www.mobimotherhood .org. Milk supply dropping, or the perception that it is, can also be misinterpreted as a sign of self-weaning. How a mother interprets and hence responds to these situations is the critical factor in ensuring milk supply continues or not. A nursing strike or a misinterpreted perception of a drop in supply can signal the end of a breastfeeding relationship and can be a very emotional time for mothers who weren't ready to finish breastfeeding. On the flip side, some mothers are ready and are at peace with whatever comes next. Should a mother wish to continue breastfeeding, then education is key to achieving this with success amid these challenges.

Premature introduction of solids: Introduction of solids too early or giving too much too soon can affect milk supply, as food may displace the need for milk, which should still be the primary food source up to 1 year of age, and in most cases, exclusively till around 6 months (see more about this in Chapter 6, "Babies and Toddlers"). A reduction in nursing due to mother or infant illness, or separation such as when babies need to be in the neonatal intensive care unit (NICU) or special care nursery (SCN) post-birth, can also reduce supply due to stress, and mostly the lack of breast contact. Similarly, separation due to work commitments can reduce supply.

Cluster feeding: There will be times, especially when it's hot or the baby is having a growth spurt, that babies feed more during the day, leaving you feeling rather drained at night (your boobs and probably your whole body!). This will often result in cluster feeding where the baby feeds in small amounts often till late evening then finally goes to sleep properly. It's important to know that the breasts will never be fully emptied, as there will always be milk available, but the baby may get cranky with the lack of flow, as it's the fatty hind milk they have to work hard to get when they cluster feed in the evenings. And though the volume they drink may be less, it's more satisfying and high calorie, so it's good for weight gain and good for a subsequent nice deep sleep.

Bottle feeding: If a bottle is given to the baby for the early evening or for late feed to supplement low supply, its best that it's a bottle of expressed milk from earlier in the day when supply is more abundant. Babies will often feed off just one full breast in the morning, so the other can be expressed and both should fill up again by the next feed. Ideally, the bottle should be given by the father (or significant other) so the baby doesn't get confused when Mama, who usually whips booby out, isn't doing so. Alternatively, you can increase the consumption of lactogenic foods from lunchtime, such as a lactation-promoting smoothies found later in this chapter!

Breast pumping: A perception of low supply can be when expressing, particularly months down the track when your response to the pump is not what it was in the early days. Pumping a small volume is not necessarily a reflection on your supply—the baby just does a much better job at stimulating let down and extracting the milk. For instance, the baby can be capable of sucking 50ml to100ml (2 to 4 ounces) in less than 10 minutes, but it could take 20 to 30 minutes to pump an ounce. If pumping is needed because you are returning to work or for other reasons, and you want to keep breastfeeding, then strategies such as heat and/or massage prior to and during pumping may help, as well as consuming lactogenic smoothies. An electric medical-grade pump will also do a better job than a battery-operated one. Also, ensure your breast shield is the correct size, as this can affect the efficiency of the suction, and the size required can change as your breasts change over time.

Softer breasts: Another perception of reduced milk supply can be found with changes around the 3- to 4-month mark. First, your breasts will be softer when they are full. Early on it is more obvious that your breasts empty and fill up, and when full can be quite firm and may be uncomfortable. However, being less obviously full is not a sign your supply is dropping: It's normal. Around this time, the baby is also more efficient at feeding and may take as little as 3 to 5 minutes per boob to feed. Mothers often stress that the baby isn't getting enough as they have not nursed for very long, but again this is quite normal. After further discussion with mothers who feel their milk supply has slowed, it is apparent that they believe their milk is a problem because their breasts are softer, and their babies are cranky and not sleeping as well, so they feel the need to add a bottle or two of formula and/or solids into the baby's diet. We know that the softening of breasts is normal, and around this age, babies are entering a huge developmental leap that sees a big change in behavior—with more crying, fussing, being clingy and regression of sleep quality (look up the "Wonder Weeks" online for more on this). This is usually age related and is unlikely due to milk supply genuinely dropping or the need to start solids.

If your baby is consistently gaining weight, is active, looks well, has plenty of wet and dirty diapers, then they are getting enough milk. If these factors are not the case, then there may be a genuine loss of supply requiring a multifaceted approach that includes ensuring there is frequent nursing and/or pumping, that you and your baby are getting enough sleep, and that you are utilizing relaxation strategies regularly. In addition, galactagogues may be used.

*Breastfeeding is something I was determined to do since
becoming pregnant with my first baby. Apart from the extremely
special bonding experience it creates between mother and child,
I know that the health benefits for the baby are immense and
it is the very best start in life a mother can give her baby—and
of course I only want the very best for my son. I also know it
is important that while my baby is receiving the best from his
mother that I am also taking care of myself nutritionally too.
Around the 6-week mark my son was feeding A LOT, which
caused me stress that my supply might be dropping. I started
drinking smoothies in my diet each day that support milk
production, and noticed a huge increase in my supply and my
energy levels. I would make a big batch in the morning and keep
it in the fridge to sip on throughout the day. I have since learned
that I have a smaller breast storage capacity than most women,
which means my bub will always feed a lot more frequently than
most other babies. If I ever feel that my supply needs a little
extra boost, especially during a growth spurt or illness, I know
I can whip a smoothie up in no time, full of milk-supportive
ingredients like oats, flax, brewer's yeast, almonds, bananas, and
coconut and notice the effects of it almost instantly! —Hilary*

Increasing Breast Milk Supply

Galactagogues are substances that are "lactogenic" and claim
to promote breast milk production in regards to flow, volume,
or release (let down). There are numerous herbs and foods that
claim to be lactogenic, based upon traditional and historical
uses. Medications can also be prescribed for this purpose. If you
have a genuine loss of supply, or are at risk of losing supply due

to separation from your baby (cessation of night feeds, returning to work, baby in hospital, etc.), then having a lactogenic diet and consuming lactogenic smoothies is a good idea. However, this must be in combination with milk being removed from the breast frequently and effectively by the baby and/or a pump; otherwise it will still be a battle to increase supply. If you look at recommended foods for a lactogenic diet generally, you will notice it is really a whole-foods, plant-based diet—with high fiber and mineral-rich whole grains, legumes, nuts, seeds, high fiber and iron-rich fruits, herbs, spices, high-antioxidant vegetables, and greens, which is probably why women who eat this way anyway are less likely to report issues with their milk supply. The functions of galactagogues are varied and ultimately act upon the hormonal system, such as stimulation of prolactin for milk volume, oxytocin production for milk ejection, stimulation of mammary tissue, and hormone balance via a healthy liver. Moreover, many galactagogues have multiple lactogenic qualities.

GALACTAGOGUES

Dopamine Suppression

Many vegetables and leafy greens help to increase prolactin via the naturally occurring opiates and dopamine-suppressing substances they contain. Suppression of dopamine facilitates the release of prolactin from the pituitary gland. Tryptophan is an amino acid that is a precursor to one of our good mood hormones, serotonin. Serotonin suppresses dopamine, and lowered dopamine means more prolactin, which in turn means more milk.

Smoothie-friendly sources of dopamine suppression: spinach, Swiss chard, kale and other brassicas, romaine lettuce, fennel tops, beet greens

Smoothie-friendly sources of tryptophan: oats, dates, dairy, eggs, tahini, sunflower seeds, pumpkin seeds, raw cacao, almonds, fennel, celery, apricot, lettuce, carrot, bananas, spinach, kale, collards, and peanuts

Minerals and B Vitamins

Most galactagogues are mineral rich, particularly with calcium, iron, magnesium, and zinc. Calcium and magnesium work together for a healthy nervous system and for correct muscle function, both helping muscles to contract and relax, and are part of the biology of milk ejection. They combat depression, anxiety, and problems sleeping, all of which interfere with milk supply. Of all nuts and seeds, almonds and sesame are considered the most lactogenic due to their high-calcium content. Similarly, the most lactogenic fruits are apricots, figs, and dates—all of which are smoothie-friendly ingredients.

Zinc requirements are high for pregnant and lactating mothers, not only for the child but also for maternal health, supporting mental health, growth, healing, and immunity.

Iron, in combination with vitamins B6, B12, and folic acid are "blood building," which in Traditional Chinese Medicine (TCM) is an essential process in the postnatal period, particularly if there has been blood loss during the birth.

Smoothie-friendly and blood-building foods: leafy greens, beets, apricots, avocado, dates, prunes, citrus, figs, nuts and seeds, blackstrap molasses, eggs, brewer's yeast, bananas, dairy products, cardamom, alfalfa, ginger, licorice, and whole grains such as quinoa and oats. TCM also advises eating the following foods to improve "qi" or "life force": oats, rice, cinnamon, clove, fennel, ginger, and nutmeg.

Phytoestrogens

We know already that estrogens have a powerful role in breast growth and development. Estrogen affects mammary growth indirectly via prolactin and growth hormone, and directly on the breast tissue itself. Dietary phytoestrogens (plant-based estrogens) and environmental xenoestrogens can alter the function of estrogen produced by the body. Environmental xenoestrogens come from plastics and chemicals in pollution and are not beneficial to the body in any way, potentially creating estrogen dominance disorders, as discussed in Chapter 3, "Making Babies."

Plant-based estrogens may be strong in effect, such as those from soy (which is not recommended), or much milder, such as those found in many foods.

Smoothie-friendly phytoestrogen foods: alfalfa, anise, apple, cabbage, carrot, cherry, dates, fennel, flax, licorice, oats, pomegranate, sesame, strawberry, and sunflower seeds

Saponins

Chemically, saponins are a "glycoside" with a soapy, bitter quality to them. They exist in plants as a defense mechanism to predators in the wild, as they taste unpleasant. In small quantities they may be beneficial, though in large amounts they will cause gastrointestinal upset, particularly bloating. Saponins coat quinoa and are also present in oats and spinach. They are believed to influence the pituitary to produce hormones of lactation. Saponins found in oats and spinach also increase and accelerate the body's ability to absorb calcium, which we know is necessary also for lactation, and both are excellent smoothie ingredients.

Liver Boosters

A healthy liver is necessary for a healthy gut and healthy hormones. Antioxidants such as glutathione, glucosinolates, chlorophyll, and carotenoids are essential for excellent liver function.

Smoothie-friendly and liver-boosting ingredients: green leafy veg (especially brassicas), carrots, beets, lemon, limes, avocado, ginger, and turmeric

Anethol

"Anethol" is the aromatic compound in fennel, anise, and licorice, which has sedating/relaxing properties. Relaxation increases oxytocin production and oxytocin is responsible for the let-down reflex. These herbs, especially fennel, also help to relax the gut, which makes a good digestive aid for mothers, and for the baby via breast milk, which may be useful for colicky babies. In smoothies, cooled tea or fresh fennel juice may be used as the liquid base, ground fennel seeds may be added, or raw fennel tops may be included. Pieces of fennel bulb are very fibrous raw and aren't very pleasant added to smoothies.

Fats

Fats are an essential component of breast milk, with around 50 percent of calories coming from fat, with lauric acid and capric acids the predominant fats. These fats are also present in coconut oil—considered a lactogenic food. In smoothies, coconut products, including cream, milk, water, and fresh flesh from drinking coconuts, are fantastic lactogenic additions.

Key Lactogenic Foods

It becomes clear that certain foods feature frequently in the various categories of galactagogues, and some are considered the key lactogenic foods to consume if milk supply is waning. These include:

- Oats

- Spinach

- Fennel

- Flax

- Brewer's yeast

- Blackstrap molasses

- Sunflower seeds

- Almonds

- Tahini

- Coconut

- Carrots

- Beets

- Leafy greens

- Apricots

- Dates

- Eggs

A popular postpartum snack for milk supply is the "lactation cookie." There are numerous variations in recipes, though the three key ingredients are oats, flax meal, and brewer's yeast. These are combined with butter, sugar, vanilla, eggs, and dried fruit such as apricots and dates or seeds such as sunflower. Some recipes use ground fennel seed, blackstrap molasses, and/or cinnamon, and coconut oil could be used instead of butter. It is suggested to eat a cookie with each breastfeed or have as a snack between main meals—the former results in eating a lot of cookies and will likely add many calories more to your diet than is needed! Alternatively, try drinking the Lactation Cookie Smoothie on page 221.

Lactogenic Teas, Powders, and Tinctures

Fenugreek is well known as a curry spice and is frequently recommended to help boost milk supply, often in combination with blessed thistle. Caution should be taken with fenugreek, because at the dosages recommended they can cause an upset tummy (for both mother and baby), reduce blood sugar, and reduce thyroid function. Furthermore, it can stimulate contractions of the uterus, and hence it is contraindicated in pregnancy (except at the end if nothing is happening and you are told to eat a curry—this is why!), and conceiving while breastfeeding is certainly possible. So if you have coexisting medical conditions such as allergies, an underactive thyroid, or diabetes, it is not wise to take it, or only under supervision of an appropriate health professional. Goat's rue, alfalfa, anise, ashwagandha, astragalus, burdock, red raspberry leaf, nettle, marshmallow root, shatavari, lemon verbena, and borage are further examples of herbs that claim to boost milk supply. These can be used as smoothie liquid bases or just drunk as teas. Goat's rue needs to be used with caution due to similar effects to fenugreek. Herbal remedies should not be self-prescribed but rather taken under the guidance of an herbalist or naturopath. Used in excess they can have the opposite of the desired effect.

Medication

Domperidone (Motilium) and metoclopramide (Maxolon) are medications that are used to treat gastrointestinal disorders but have also been shown to increase milk supply. They act by blocking dopamine, which is a hormone that inhibits prolactin release. These medications can have unpleasant side effects and should only be used under medical supervision and ideally as a last resort.

Foods and Drinks to Avoid While Breastfeeding

Foods such as refined sugar, coffee, and alcohol rob nutrients from the body, have taxing effects on the liver, cause oxidative stress (formation of free radicals), and elevate stress hormones that restrict blood vessels in the breasts impairing let down—so all are best avoided while breastfeeding. Furthermore, medications such as antihistamines, diuretics, and decongestants can negatively influence milk supply. Consumed in large quantities, lemon balm, parsley, rosemary, peppermint, spearmint, sage, and thyme are documented as being anti-lactogenic. Just to confuse matters, small amounts are considered beneficial for their rich mineral and antioxidant content, so enjoy these herbs for culinary purposes in moderation and avoid in excess.

Since I knew I was going to be separated from my baby immediately post-birth, and I had to have a C-section, both of which pose risks to building and maintaining milk supply once the milk comes in (due to stress, and lack of breast- and skin-to-skin contact), I used every trick in the book. I baked lactation cookies before I went into the hospital and took some with me to start eating for a healthy milk supply post-birth. I drank coconut water, carrot and beet juice, green smoothies and fennel tea, took fenugreek and blessed thistle tablets, and I expressed at least 8 times a day. I may have gone overboard but it still took a good 6 to 8 weeks for my milk supply to get where it needed to be. I always had enough for my baby as she was little and on measured volumes of milk according to her weight. In the end I had oversupply and it took till we had been home 4 to 6 weeks for this to balance out, expressing for my comfort and for my daughter's, to avoid an overload of lactose-rich foremilk.

In my time visiting the NICU/SCN where my baby stayed for 8 weeks, I got to know many mothers, some of whom struggled with their milk supply—if not at first, further down the track. A key observation I made was rather poor dietary choices, with fast foods, sweets, coffee, and colas being consumed on a regular basis, not to mention mothers that were smokers. Lactation consultants were great at supporting pumping technique and breastfeeding when it could begin, but little was ever mentioned about diet and lifestyle, and medication was the next port of call, which often didn't work, as the mother had got too stressed and wasn't pumping often enough anymore for enough prolactin to be stimulated. Thanks to my obsession with ensuring I had enough milk, I was, according to the head lactation consultant in the NICU, an absolute rarity, given my baby was exclusively fed breast milk without any supplementation ever. There is no moral high ground I stand upon over my achievements, as the unusual outcome shocked me. I just did what I knew had to be done with the knowledge I had. My daughter was fortunate I had this knowledge and the motivation. It wasn't easy: It was really hard work, but well worth it.

Food Intolerances and Allergies While Breastfeeding

The digestive system of a baby is not mature at birth, nor for the first 6 or so months when the gut is "open," meaning the spaces that allow nutrients to move from the gut into the bloodstream are large enough to allow immune supportive antibodies from breast milk through. They will also allow food particles through, with dairy foods as the number-one food likely to causes problems, followed by other protein foods such as eggs, soy, gluten, tree nuts, and groundnuts (peanuts), as well as synthetic chemical additives, and also natural chemicals in healthy foods such as amines, salicylates, and glutamate. Furthermore, anything that makes mother gassy may make baby gassy. When you list all the potential foods that could be a problem it's a ridiculously long list, so it is not advised to avoid anything while breastfeeding simply out of caution. It's important for a mother's nutrition to eat a varied diet, and it is believed that when a baby is exposed to varied foods via breast milk (as food will alter the flavor—especially things like garlic, spices, and vanilla), babies are more likely to accept a varied diet when solids are introduced.

Human milk's primary carbohydrate is lactose, which provides 40 percent of the milk's energy. This amount is the highest of all mammalian milks, making it the sweetest. Lactose helps calcium and iron be absorbed, and there is also an abundance of the enzyme lactase in breast milk to help digest it. Both human milk and cow's milk contain lactose and the milk protein, casein. It should be noted that a baby cannot be allergic to its mother's milk—the baby may be intolerant to high levels of lactose if getting too much foremilk, the lactose-rich, watery milk that comes out of the breast at the start of a feed (typical of women with oversupply with baby not draining the breast per feed), or they may be allergic to particles in breast milk from the mother's diet. If there is a reaction to dairy foods by the baby via the breast milk, it is to the cow's milk casein. If a dairy intolerance is suspected in a baby, then cow's milk or yogurt should not be used in smoothies consumed by the breastfeeding mother. Cow's milk protein is the most common cause of allergy-related upsets in babies. Only small amounts of milk may be ingested in things like warm drinks; however, larger quantities may be consumed in smoothies—but both large and small amounts should be avoided till breastfeeding ceases.

If you find you have a particularly unsettled baby with reflux, vomiting, colic, severe fussing, poor sleep, and/or abnormal bowel habits, or there are visual signs such as eczema, rashes, or wheezing, then considering a source of irritation via the mother's diet is worthwhile. If either parent—and especially both—has food intolerances or allergies, then the risk of their baby having them too are increased as there is a genetic component to allergies. Problems with eggs and dairy are frequently grown out of with time, but things like gluten and nuts are not.

Given that the predominant potential irritant is dairy, this is the most logical one to eliminate to see if anything changes. If multiple foods are suspected and you don't have a very good knowledge of nutrition, then it's wise to do elimination and reintroduction under the guidance of a health professional who specializes in this field. If a baby has allergy testing (such as skin prick testing) that reveals positive reactions, then these foods, unless advised otherwise, should not be consumed by the breastfeeding mother because the allergenic proteins are passed to baby via the breast milk. This can mean not using ingredients like eggs, nut milks and butters, and/or dairy in smoothies. If all cannot be consumed, then being more creative with elements that make smoothies nice and creamy is required. Frozen bananas are extra creamy, sunflower seeds are good instead of eggs, since they're rich in choline, and avocados and coconut products will be your best friends!

My daughter had eczema on her arms, legs, and chest, which wasn't clearing with various moisturizers or the removal of dairy foods. But when I stopped eggs, it cleared up completely, as did her tendency to have a lot of nasal boogers and fussing during and after feed times. Allergy testing subsequently revealed allergies to eggs, cashews, and almonds, which meant none of these were allowed in my diet and smoothies anymore while breastfeeding.

My son was not gaining any weight as a newborn and fell below birth weight at 3 months old. I worked with a homeopath/ naturopath who took me off salicylates, amines, and acid foods. I also lost weight and was close to 40kg, which clearly didn't help either of us. The sensitivities were blurred because I became stressed, which affected my mind, body, and spirit. With me being unwell, I had to get myself better and my son better, so unfortunately we breastfeed no longer after 8 months. His first solid food was pear and rice for at least 12 months, and then we gradually introduced low-acid foods. —Caroline

My third munchkin had a dairy allergy that resulted in bloody stools when I ate dairy. I went dairy-free for 18 months until he tested clear of the allergy. He continued to nurse for another few months with no problems, though I never went back to dairy as fully as I had been prior. —Sandy

The Smoothies

The recipes in this chapter can all be considered supportive of breast milk supply (or lactogenic) by default, given they are full of whole foods rich in antioxidants, good fats, minerals, and vitamins.

Some, however, are designed to be more lactogenic than others, and these can be used in situations with a genuine drop in milk supply or a risk of a drop in milk supply due to separation from the baby at birth, illness of mother or baby, high stress, major sleep deprivation, drop in night feeds, returning to work, etc. Once supply is restored, go back to the regular smoothies, since otherwise there is a chance of oversupply and risks the development of blocked ducts and mastitis, plus an overload of lactose-rich foremilk received by your baby, which may upset their gut, especially if they don't drain the breast and balance it out with the fattier hindmilk. This may also occur if you falsely believe your supply is dropping per the examples already discussed. If you do find yourself in this situation with breasts that are getting engorged, then express some milk for comfort (with a pump or manually) prior to a feed and back off with the consumption of stronger galactagogues.

Recipes in this chapter make approximately 500ml/2 cups, which is a large serving for one or two smaller servings. The exception is the Highly Lactogenic Smoothies (page 220), which make 1 liter (4 cups). Smoothies may be consumed for breakfast like I have them, or they can be any meal of the day, or even a snack. Whenever they suit you to have them, consider if your partner (if you have one) will have some too, or if you have other children you may share it with. If more than 2 cups of a smoothie are needed, simply double the recipe. Sharing a lactogenic smoothie with someone not breastfeeding is not a problem either, as they are simply extra nutritious and won't make them start lactating! Furthermore, if you are not breastfeeding, drinking smoothies designed to promote or support lactation won't make you start to lactate either, because the key factor with milk production is nipple suckling by a baby (or breast pump). Instead, the recipes will provide plenty of nutrients to support your energy and stress levels, and immune system—all of which need support when you are a mother (and father!).

According to my survey, 63 percent of mothers drinking smoothies while pregnant and breastfeeding did not change the content of their smoothie compared to their usual pre-pregnancy recipes. Given nutrient requirements are different and more demanding during these times, it is wise to make them more nutritious than usual, particularly if the typical smoothie is just milk and a banana—not that this isn't nutritious, but it can be better.

Postnatally, eggs can again be consumed in smoothies. There isn't anything specifically off the smoothie menu when breastfeeding except to be careful with anything stimulating like cacao, and drinking tea or coffee. These three are often a savior for sleep-deprived mamas to give them a lift; however, if the baby is stimulated by these via breast milk then adapt your intake according. If thyroid health is an issue, then avoid the recipes containing goitrogenic ingredients or make substitutions for other similar ingredients: swap kale for Swiss chard, swap peanut butter for almond butter, swap peaches for apricots, etc.

Should you be breastfeeding and you have been advised to eliminate foods from your diet that you or your baby are sensitive to, then the following are suggested substitutions:

SUGGESTED SUBSTITUTIONS

INSTEAD OF	USE
Dairy yogurt	Coconut yogurt
Dairy milk	Nut or seed milk, coconut milk, coconut water, or water
Nuts (general)	Seeds such as sunflower, pumpkin, hemp, or sesame (tahini), or dairy or coconut milk in place of nut milk
Almonds	Tahini (for reasons of calcium), cashew, or macadamia (for more similar flavor)
Cashews	Macadamias or hemp seeds (for creaminess)
Peanuts	Almonds or sunflower seeds
Eggs	1 tablespoon each of sunflower seeds and chia seeds or ground flax—to supply omegas, protein, and choline
Brassicas such as kale, cabbage, bok choy	Spinach, beet leaves, Swiss chard, butter or romaine lettuce, mint, parsley

Please note that recipes will vary in thickness and sweetness according to the choice of ingredients and this will vary further, particularly with flavor, due to differences between seasons and produce quality. Should a recipe turn out thicker than you would like, add some more liquid; if it's not sweet enough, add some sweetener; if you like cold smoothies, use some ice in place of the liquid component. If you haven't read the introductory chapters before attempting my recipes, please go back and read them, particularly Chapter 1, "The Art and Science of Smoothies," which has detailed guidelines for my smoothie creations.

In addition, all recipe titles marked with a carrot (🥕) in this chapter refer to recipes that match a smoothie base recipe for babies, which will be explained in the baby and toddler recipe section.

THE FIRST 6 WEEKS

Immediately after birth and the first 6 weeks is a time for rest and recovery. You will be learning all about your new baby, as well as needing plenty of time for healing and reduced swelling from pregnancy. Nutrients required to nourish during this time include protein, fats, vitamins A, C, and E, biotin, silica, and zinc, as well as plenty of cleansing leafy greens, and calories to satisfy increased appetite.

🥕 Sweet Satisfaction

½ cup steamed or pureed sweet potato or pumpkin

1 banana, fresh or frozen and sliced

1 tablespoon peanut butter or heaped tablespoon of sunflower seeds*

¼ inch sliced fresh ginger

½ teaspoon ground turmeric

pinch of nutmeg

1 cup almond milk

1–2 handfuls of spinach (optional)

*Ideally, soak seeds overnight in water, then drain and rinse before use.

3Bs: Banana, Beets, and Berries

1 banana, fresh or frozen and sliced

¼ cup diced raw or steamed beet

1 cup frozen blueberries

¾ cup any milk

10 raw cashews

1–2 Swiss chard leaves (optional)

Love Those Legs Again

1 Persian cucumber, quartered

1½ cups watermelon

3 sprigs mint leaves

Gimme a Boost

1 banana, frozen and sliced

1 serving of plant-based protein powder

½ teaspoon vanilla extract or paste, or ¼ vanilla bean

1 cup any milk

1 heaping teaspoon raw cacao plus tiny pinch of salt (optional)

Waldorf Wonderland

1 rib of celery, chopped into 1-inch pieces

1 packed cup seedless grapes

½ cup dairy or almond milk

1 heaping tablespoon walnuts or pecans*

4 ice cubes

sweeten to taste

*Ideally, soak overnight, drain, and rinse before blending—this will aid digestion as well as improve the strong flavor of the walnuts once blended.

Sustaining Strawberries

1½ cups/1 punnet strawberries with hulls

1 tablespoon ground flaxseed

¼ cup natural yogurt plus ½ cup milk, or ¾ cup milk kefir

3 medjool dates, pitted

3 ice cubes

Coco-Banana Passion

1 large banana, frozen and sliced

baby bok choy (optional), trimmed and well washed

½ cup coconut flesh and ¾ cup coconut water from a drinking coconut

pulp of 1 passion fruit*

*Blend all except passion fruit, which you stir through at the end by hand.

Apricot Tart

1 banana, fresh or frozen and sliced

½ cup peach or apricot halves, fresh* or steamed

¼ teaspoon ground Sri Lankan cinnamon

1 cup coconut water

1 egg (optional)

*It's essential that fresh stone fruit are ripe, sweet, and juicy.

Raspberry Rehabilitation

1½ cups frozen raspberries

10 raw cashews

1 serving plant-based protein powder

1 cup coconut water

5–6 butter lettuce leaves or 2–3 romaine lettuce leaves (optional)

Papaya and Mango Mender

¾ cup papaya

¾ cup mango flesh

¾ cup coconut water

2 tablespoons hemp seeds

1 teaspoon vanilla extract or paste, or ½ vanilla bean

1 egg (optional)

1–2 handfuls of spinach (optional)

STRESS-BUSTING SMOOTHIES

The postnatal period can be a very stressful time for many new mothers, particularly if the baby is unsettled or Mama is sleep deprived. Eating nutrient-dense foods, especially those that are good for boosting mood, busting stress, and supporting the adrenals, are essential and include saturated fats, zinc, B6, folate, B12, vitamin C, tyrosine, tryptophan, and licorice root.

. . . .

Banana and Protein Punch

1 banana, fresh or frozen and sliced

¼ avocado

1 serving plant-based protein powder

1 cup coconut water

1 teaspoon vanilla extract or paste, or ½ vanilla bean

. . . .

Sunny Strawberries and Cream

2 tablespoons raw oats plus ½ cup milk, or ½ cup porridge

1½ cups/1 punnet strawberries with hulls

¼ cup full-fat natural yogurt plus ¼ cup any milk, or ½ cup milk kefir

3 medjool dates, pitted

pulp of 1 passion fruit*

*Blend all except passion fruit, which you stir through at the end by hand.

Peaceful Papaya

1 packed cup papaya

¼ cup coconut flesh and ¾ cup coconut water from a drinking coconut

¼ inch slice fresh ginger

1 bulb baby bok choy (optional), trimmed and well washed

Cheerful Cherries

1 banana, fresh or frozen and sliced

1 cup pitted cherries

¾ cup any milk or water

10 raw cashews

1–2 handfuls of spinach (optional)

Spicy Sweet Potato

½ cup steamed or pureed sweet potato or pumpkin

¾ cup mango flesh

2 tablespoons hemps seeds

¼ teaspoon ground Sri Lankan cinnamon

pinch of ground nutmeg

pinch of ground cloves

1 cup any milk

Fig and Ginger Fun

1 banana, frozen and sliced

3 fresh figs, stem tips removed

1 serving plant-based protein powder

¼ teaspoon ground Sri Lankan cinnamon

thin slice of fresh ginger

1 cup almond milk

handful of butter lettuce (optional)

Fun with Fennel

1½ cups beet and fennel juice

1–2 handfuls of fennel tops

8 raw macadamias

1 tablespoon chia seeds

4 ice cubes

Banana Choc Content

2 bananas, fresh or frozen and sliced

1 heaping teaspoon raw cacao plus a tiny pinch of salt

1 tablespoon pumpkin seeds*

1 tablespoon hulled tahini

¾ cup coconut water

2 medjool dates, pitted

2–3 sprigs mint leaves (optional)

*Ideally, soak seeds overnight in water, then drain and rinse before use.

🥕 Merry Milky Mango

1 cup mango flesh (about 1 mango)

pinch of ground cardamom

1 heaping tablespoon sunflower seeds*

3 medjool dates, pitted

1 cup any milk

handful of Swiss chard (optional)

*Ideally, soak seeds overnight in water, then drain and rinse before use.

Absolute Refreshment

1 cup fresh pineapple pieces

1 Persian cucumber, quartered

3 ice cubes

1–2 handfuls of fennel tops

Minty Licorice Love

1 cup cooled licorice root or fennel tea

1 Granny Smith apple cut into 8 pieces or 1 pear, quartered

3 sprigs mint leaves

4 ice cubes

Breakfast Hugs

2 tablespoons raw oats plus ½ cup water or milk, or ½ cup cooked oats, quinoa, or millet

1 banana, fresh or frozen and sliced

1 tablespoon blackstrap molasses

1 cup any milk

1–2 handfuls of spinach (optional)

1 egg (optional)

SMOOTHIES FOR BREAST MILK QUALITY

Breast milk quality can be influenced by diet, with omega-3 DHA and vitamins B12, C, and D being the most significant for the mother to consume. Also important are vitamins A, E, and K, iodine, manganese, zinc, and probiotics. Probiotic supplements may be added to all recipes except those with kefir or kombucha, which are beverages containing probiotics already. With the exception of vitamin D and DHA, the remaining ingredients can be included in smoothies below.

Vitamin Virtue

1 cup fresh pineapple

1 kiwi with skin, halved

¼ lime (flesh and peel)

¾ cup coconut water

3 ice cubes

3 sprigs mint leaves

Pear and Peanut Potion

2 tablespoons raw oats plus ½ cup water or milk, or ½ cup cooked oats, quinoa, or millet

2 pears, quartered

1 tablespoon peanut butter

¾ cup almond milk

3 ice cubes

1 egg (optional)

Apricot and Macadamia Marvel

1 mixed cup nectarine and apricot halves*

1 cup coconut water

6 raw macadamias

thin slice of fresh ginger

1 teaspoon vanilla extract or paste, or ½ vanilla bean

1 bulb baby bok choy (optional), trimmed and well washed

*It's essential that fresh stone fruit are ripe, sweet, and juicy.

Berry and Banana Blessings

1 banana

1 cup frozen berries

¼ avocado

¾ cup any milk

1 egg (optional)

1–2 handfuls of spinach (optional)

Fennel and Turmeric Tincture

1 cup fresh pineapple pieces

1 banana, fresh or frozen and sliced

½ teaspoon ground turmeric

handful of fennel tops or 1 teaspoon ground fennel*

¾ cup any milk

10 raw cashews or 5 macadamias

1 egg (optional)

*Grind fennel seeds with a spice grinder or mortar and pestle.

Spectacular Strawberries

1 cup papaya

1½ cups/1 punnet strawberries with hulls

2 tablespoons hemp seeds

pulp of 1 passion fruit*

*Blend all except passion fruit, which you stir through at the end by hand.

Kombucha and Melon Marvel

1 cup watermelon

1 cup honeydew melon

½ cup kombucha*

*Aim for low-sugar varieties; this not an appropriate ingredient to share with an infant.

🥕 Spiced Pumpkin and Banana Brew

½ cup steamed or pureed sweet potato or pumpkin

1 banana, fresh or frozen and sliced

¼ cup natural yogurt plus ¾ cup milk, or 1 cup milk kefir

¼ teaspoon ground Sri Lankan cinnamon

½ teaspoon ground turmeric

pinch of ground cloves

pinch of ground nutmeg

1 egg (optional)

sweeten to taste

handful of butter or romaine lettuce (optional)

IMMUNE-BOOSTING SMOOTHIES

Trying to maintain a strong immune system can be difficult as a new mother, particularly if sleep deprived and being "too busy" to eat and drink properly. The following immune-boosting smoothies contain vitamins A, C, and E, B vitamins, iodine, selenium, zinc, manganese, and probiotics. Probiotic supplements may be added to all recipes except those with kefir or kombucha, which are beverages containing probiotics already.

🥕 Papaya and Lime Lift

¾ cup papaya

1 banana, fresh or frozen and sliced

juice of ½ lime

¼ cup coconut flesh and ¾ cup coconut water from a drinking coconut

1 egg (optional)

Summer Love

¾ cup mango flesh

¾ cup peach halves*

¾ cup any milk

1 teaspoon vanilla extract or paste, or ½ vanilla bean

10 raw cashews

1 egg (optional)

2–3 romaine lettuce leaves (optional)

*It's essential that stone fruit is ripe, sweet, and juicy.

Melon and Passion Fruit Pleasure

1 cup cantaloupe

1 cup honeydew melon

1 tablespoon chia seeds

1–2 Swiss chard leaves (optional)

pulp of 1 passion fruit*

*Blend all except passion fruit, which you stir through at the end by hand.

Selenium Salvation

¾ cup nectarine halves*

¾ cup pineapple, fresh or small frozen pieces

¾ cup coconut water

4 Brazil nuts**

4–6 butter lettuce leaves (optional)

*It's essential that the nectarines are ripe, sweet, and juicy.

**Ideally, soak seeds overnight in water, then drain and rinse before use.

Pineapple and Turmeric Tonic

1 cup pineapple, fresh or small frozen pieces

¼ avocado

½ teaspoon ground turmeric

pinch of nutmeg

1 cup almond milk

1–2 handfuls of spinach (optional)

1 egg (optional)

Probiotic Punch

¾ cup frozen blueberries

1 banana

¼ cup natural yogurt plus ¾ cup milk, or 1 cup milk kefir

1 heaping tablespoon sunflower, pumpkin seeds, or mixture*

1 egg (optional)

sweeten to taste

2–3 kale or Chinese cabbage leaves (optional)

*Ideally, soak seeds overnight in water, then drain and rinse before use.

More Than a Juice

1 cup beet and carrot juice

1½ cups/1 punnet strawberries with hulls

1 tablespoon chia seeds

This smoothie will be thin to start with and will thicken as the chia swells up.

Antioxidant Advantage

1 cup pitted cherries

½ cup pomegranate juice*

½ cup coconut milk

1 tablespoon chia seeds

3 ice cubes

handful of parsley (optional)

2 tablespoons pomegranate seeds (optional) **

*To juice pomegranates, blend the seeds for 10–15 seconds then strain through a fine sieve.

**If using a fresh pomegranate, reserve some seeds before juicing the rest.

HIGHLY LACTOGENIC SMOOTHIES

A diet rich in a variety of whole foods will contain "galactagogues" that help to improve breast milk quantity. If your diet is not rich in whole foods and/or your milk supply is waning, then the following ingredients are the key galactagogues to consume in smoothies.

• Grains: oats, quinoa

• Nuts: peanuts, Brazil nuts, almonds

• Seeds: flax, chia, sunflower, hemp, tahini

• Veg: carrots, beets, green leafy vegetables, especially spinach, fennel

• Fruit: apricots, bananas, figs, citrus, avocado

• Other: brewer's yeast, coconut, dates, eggs, blackstrap molasses, ginger, dairy

   The following recipes are designed for mothers with a genuine reduction in breast milk who wish to increase it again. Please ensure your supply is truly low, otherwise you risk oversupply—see the discussion earlier in this chapter that covers perceived versus actual drop in supply. Furthermore, these highly lactogenic smoothie recipes must be paired with frequent removal of milk from the breast to work. The base recipe is based upon the lactation cookie with variations suggested. These recipes make around 1 liter/4 cups (4 servings) and I suggest drinking a cup as a snack 4 times a day (not unlike eating a lactation cookie semi-regularly). If you mostly struggle with supply at the end of each day, you could also try drinking smoothies in the afternoon only. Each recipe was tested by me or another breastfeeding mama with all of us reporting increased supply as a result.

Two recipes call for carrot juice and though it takes some planning, it's worth it, as it tastes much nicer than whole carrot. If you have a juicer, make the most of getting it out of the cupboard and make plenty of juice. It will last a few days in the fridge, or freeze portions and thaw them out as needed. Alternatively, ask a helpful friend with a juicer to make some for you.

Lactation Cookie Smoothie Base Recipe

1½ cups dairy or almond milk

4 tablespoons raw oats plus ¾ cup water or milk, or 1 cup porridge

1 tablespoon brewer's yeast

2 tablespoons ground flaxseed

2 eggs

2 teaspoons vanilla extract or paste, or 1 vanilla bean, halved

1 teaspoon ground cinnamon

2 bananas, fresh or frozen and sliced

4 medjool dates, pitted

Variations on the base recipe:

- Substitute cooked quinoa or cooked millet for oats
- Add a tablespoon of blackstrap molasses
- Substitute maple syrup for dates
- Substitute coconut milk for dairy or almond
- Substitute chia seeds for flax or use a combination of both
- Substitute carrot juice for milk
- Substitute "nursing tea" for milk
- Add more spices, including any or all of
  - ¼ teaspoon ground cardamom
  - 1 teaspoon ground turmeric
  - ½-inch piece fresh ginger
  - 2 teaspoons ground fennel seeds
- Use more fat, such as
  - 2 tablespoons peanut butter or tahini
  - 3 tablespoons sunflower, hemp, or pumpkin seeds
  - ½ avocado
- Substitute soaked, dried figs or apricots for bananas
- Add some leafy greens, especially spinach

Milk-Making Machine

½ cup diced raw beet

½ cup pomegranate juice*

1 packed cup fresh cherries

flesh and water from 1 drinking coconut

2 handfuls of beet greens or parsley

6 ice cubes

*To juice pomegranates yourself, blend the seeds for 10–15 seconds then strain through a fine sieve. Alternatively, you can buy commercially prepared pomegranate juice at your convenience, but please ensure it is 100 percent pomegranate, with no added sugar.

Vitamin and Mineral Miracle

4 tablespoons raw oats plus 6 dried figs, soaked in 3 cups any milk overnight in the fridge

2 tablespoons blackstrap molasses

1 tablespoon Brewer's yeast

6 ice cubes

1–2 eggs (optional)

This is a strong-tasting smoothie (thanks to the molasses) but very delicious, and contains three of the stronger galactagogues: oats, molasses, and brewer's yeast.

Molasses Monster

4 tablespoons raw oats plus ¾ cup milk or water, or 1 cup cooled porridge

2 bananas, fresh or frozen and sliced

4 medjool dates, pitted

1½ cups any milk

1–2 eggs

2–3 handfuls of spinach

2 tablespoons blackstrap molasses*

*Add molasses last, otherwise it tends to sink to the bottom of the blender.

Carrot and Apricot Abundance

½ cup fresh or steamed apricot halves*

½ cup fresh or steamed peach halves

1 tablespoon hulled tahini

1 tablespoon almond butter

2 tablespoons ground flaxseed

½ inch slice fresh ginger

½ teaspoon ground Sri Lankan cinnamon

¼ teaspoon ground nutmeg

4 medjool dates, pitted

2 cups carrot juice

*It's essential that fresh apricots are ripe, sweet, and juicy.

Invisible Anethol

1½ cups orange or mandarin orange segments

flesh and zest from 1 lemon

2 cups cold sweetened fennel tea: 2 cups boiling water, 2 teaspoons
  fennel seeds, 2 teaspoons of honey

6 ice cubes

4 Chinese cabbage leaves or 2 bulbs baby bok choy

This smoothie has a consistency more like a juice and is tart from the lemon, but
pleasantly so. The zest is strong tasting so reduce to half if you prefer, but the zest
is extremely good for you, especially for the liver. Due to the lemon, the fennel
can't be tasted, so it's great for those of you who dislike fennel but would like its
benefits to milk supply and the let-down reflex. Anethol is the active essential oil
in fennel.

The Most Excellent Elixir

2 bananas, frozen and sliced

1 pear, quartered (must be soft and juicy)

2 tablespoons hulled tahini

2 cups carrot juice

1 teaspoon ground turmeric

½ inch slice fresh ginger

2 teaspoons vanilla extract or paste, or 1 vanilla bean

1 serving plant-based protein powder

½–1 tablespoon brewer's yeast (optional)

Choc-Banana Bounty

4 tablespoons raw oats plus ¾ cup water or milk, or 1 cup cooked oats, quinoa, or millet

2 bananas, fresh or frozen and sliced

1½ cups dairy or almond milk

1 tablespoon raw cacao plus pinch of salt

6 medjool dates, pitted

¼–½ inch slice fresh ginger

1 tablespoon brewer's yeast

1–2 eggs (optional)

Over a whole day, the 1 tablespoon of cacao should not pose issues as a stimulant; rather, it will be for flavor. However, if your baby is particularly sensitive to your consumption of caffeine or chocolate, then best to omit it or perhaps try carob powder.

Boobie Breakthrough

2 bananas, fresh or frozen and sliced

1½ cups pineapple

1½ cups any milk

1 teaspoon ground turmeric

2 teaspoons vanilla extract or paste, or 1 vanilla bean

2 teaspoons ground fennel*

1 cup alfalfa sprouts

2 tablespoons chia seeds or ground flaxseed

1–2 eggs (optional)

*Grind fennel seeds in a spice grinder or mortar and pestle.

If you dislike the flavor of fennel, you won't like this smoothie. Please ensure the pineapple is sweet and juicy, otherwise it will be tart and bland. If you are heartburn prone and tend to find pineapples irritating, then give this one a miss.

SMOOTHIES FOR MAINTAINING A HEALTHY MILK SUPPLY

The following smoothie recipes contain weaker galactagogues and are suitable for maintaining a healthy milk supply.

Creamy Choc-Orange

1 packed cup orange or mandarin orange segments

3 tablespoons hemp seeds

1 heaping teaspoon cacao and tiny pinch of salt

1 cup any milk

3 medjool dates, pitted

4–6 butter lettuce leaves or 2 romaine lettuce leaves (optional)

🥕 Spicy Pear and Pumpkin

½ cup steamed or pureed sweet potato or pumpkin

1 pear, quartered

1 cup any milk

¼ teaspoon ground cardamom

¼ inch slice fresh ginger

1 teaspoon vanilla extract or paste, or ½ vanilla bean

2 medjool dates, pitted

🥕 Motherly Mango

1 cup mango flesh (about 1 mango)

1 banana, fresh or frozen and sliced

¾ cup any milk

1 teaspoon vanilla extract or paste, or ½ vanilla bean

1 egg (optional)

1–2 handfuls of spinach (optional)

Overnight Smoothie

2 tablespoon raw oats

1¼ cups non-dairy milk (not coconut)

2 dried figs

2 pitted prunes

2 dried apricots

2 tablespoons hemp seeds

Combine all ingredients in a bowl in the fridge overnight, and then blend the contents the next day.

🥕 Fearless Fennel and Chocolate

2 pears, quartered (must be soft and juicy)

2 tablespoons hemp seeds

¾ cup any milk

1 heaping teaspoon raw cacao plus tiny pinch of salt

3 sprigs mint leaves

1 teaspoon ground fennel*

3 ice cubes

sweeten to taste

*Grind fennel seeds in a spice grinder or mortar and pestle.

Raspberry Remedy

2 tablespoons raw oats plus ½ cup water or milk, or ½ cup cooked oats, quinoa, or millet

¾ cup frozen raspberries

zest from ¼ lemon*

1 cup any milk

1 heaping tablespoon sunflower seeds**

3 medjool dates, pitted

*Use a vegetable peeler to remove zest.

**Ideally, soak seeds overnight in water, then drain and rinse before use.

Pineapple and Fennel Fantasy

1 cup pineapple, fresh or frozen small pieces

1 Persian cucumber, quartered

2 handfuls of fennel tops or 1 teaspoon ground fennel seeds*

5 ice cubes

*Grind in a spice grinder or mortar and pestle.

CHAPTER 6

Babies and Toddlers

At around 6 months of age, your little one can start eating and drinking foods other than breast milk or formula. This is a time of mixed emotion as your baby is growing up—and it will seem like yesterday they were born. It can be great fun introducing solids, as well as potentially stressful and definitely messy! Of most concern for parents is when to start and with what, and despite quite clear standards by organizations such as the WHO, there is great variation in advice and practice when it comes to giving food to babies, with the "why we give babies food" perhaps not taken as seriously as it needs to be—there is a lot more to it than fuel to help them grow bigger. Then there is how to do it: to spoon feed, or try baby-led weaning? And how should food, milk, naps, and play be coordinated? There is a lot to do in an older baby's day. How much do you feed them and how often? How much milk and what type of milk? How about allergies and dealing with fussy eaters? All of this I will cover and more in this chapter, including how the use of smoothies can play an important role.

Why We Introduce Solids

We eat for many reasons: for pleasure, as fuel, and for growth and repair. As babies grow, they are frequently weighed and measured, and comparisons are made to the "charts." Then if you have a big baby or a small one, it may be implied they are eating too much or too little. Questions can be incessant: How many breastfeeds or bottles? How many meals and how much volume? How about snacks? In my experience, the emphasis is always on food volume (and I count milk as food) and not food quality (the exception being the emphasis on babies from 6 months receiving enough iron from solids). Sure, volume and calories are absolutely important, but let's not forget nutrition.

As discussed in Chapter 5, "After the Baby Is Born," breast milk (or formula) supplies the ideal balance of calories, water, and nutrients for a newborn baby, and is the only food they require up to around 6 months of age. Any advice or opinion that it's pointless to continue breastfeeding beyond 6 months is wrong, and unfortunately, this can be recommended by doctors and by well-meaning, but unqualified, family and friends. Breast milk is preferable for a baby at any age in comparison to non-human milk; however, there are limited ingredients in breast milk (and formula) after 6 months, namely vitamin A, calcium, iron, and zinc—which are abundant in a varied whole-food diet. From around 6 months, infants need a combination of milk (breast or formula) and solid food to cover nutrient requirements. From a volume and calories perspective, most babies could easily be raised on breast milk or formula alone—however, they risk these key nutrient deficiencies with the absence of solid food. These deficiencies are still at risk of developing with poor choice of introduced food.

For clarity and simplicity, when I refer to "solids" this means any food or drink other than formula or breast milk. This is also known by the German word *beikost* or "complementary foods." "Solids" is simply easier to refer to.

KEY NUTRIENTS FOR BABIES AND TODDLERS

Iron

Full-term infants are born with a large store of iron, mostly in the liver and to a lesser extent in bone marrow, muscles, and the spleen. About 80 percent of iron present in a term newborn is transferred from mother to infant after 30 weeks gestation, and will be sufficient for around 6 months (unless the mother was severely anemic), when solids are introduced, and particularly iron-rich solids. Premature infants are hence born iron deficient, especially if born before 30 weeks, and will be given iron supplements. Breast milk, however, does supply some iron, and will continue to for as long as breastfeeding occurs. About 50 percent of iron in breast milk is absorbed compared to 18 percent from an omnivorous diet, 10 percent from a vegetarian diet, 7 percent in fortified formula, and 4 percent from fortified cereals. Iron requirements rise from 0.2mg per day in the first 6 months to 11mg per day in the second 6 months, and 7mg as toddlers.

Remember iron is needed to make hemoglobin, the component of red blood cells that carries oxygen around the body to its tissues and organs. Iron is marketed as being essential for brain health for babies and kids; it doesn't directly act on the brain but it is needed to ensure enough oxygen gets to the brain—and that brain is growing and developing fast! Iron deficiency may also reduce appetite, which is a double-edged sword for infants who are iron deficient and need to eat more iron-rich foods.

Given vitamin C helps with iron absorption and vitamin A helps release stored iron, a smoothie that contains these three nutrients together is sensible. Combining greens and fresh fruit to make a green smoothie will have this covered.

As previously discussed, heme iron, which comes from animal sources, is more easily absorbed than non-heme iron found in plants. Sources of heme iron are limited for smoothies, though this does include eggs. Raw eggs, many would say, should not be given to children at all; however, I know many mothers who follow the guidelines in "Fats in Smoothies" on page 21 and add raw eggs to smoothies after a child is 1 year of age.

Smoothie-friendly iron sources for children: leafy greens, especially spinach, chard, and parsley; dried apricots, figs, raspberries, raisins, prunes, beets, tahini, turmeric, pumpkin seeds, hemp seeds, quinoa, and raw eggs (for children over 1 year old)

Zinc

Zinc levels in breast milk are reduced from 4mg a liter to 1.2mg by 6 months, with the requirement from 7 months onward being 3mg. Like iron, it is required from zinc-rich foods in addition to breast milk or formula. Similarly, zinc is absorbed far more readily from breast milk than formula, which is why formula needs high amounts of iron and zinc to be effective.

Because zinc is necessary for the synthesis of all proteins in the body including genetic material, it is of paramount importance to a body that is growing, such as a child; hence, zinc deficiency may lead to stunted growth. Zinc is also important for healing, immunity, and detoxification. It is needed to convert beta-carotene from plants to the active form of vitamin A.

Smoothie-friendly zinc sources for children: coconut, cashews, Swiss chard, spinach, parsley, raw eggs (for children over 1 year old), macadamias, maple syrup, oats, pecans, peanuts, hemp seeds, pumpkin seeds, tahini, figs, ginger root, almonds, and sunflower seeds

Calcium and Vitamin D

Calcium levels in breast milk reduce by approximately 20 percent in the second 6 months of breastfeeding, and a baby's need increases by approximately 20 percent. About 270mg of calcium is required for an infant of 6 to 12 months old, and this amount jumps to 500mg for 1- to 3-year-olds. Like iron and zinc, calcium is more bioavailable from food and breast milk than from formula. The amount of calcium in breast milk from 7 to 12 months is 210mg per liter, which means 126mg is supplied based on the estimated 600ml consumed at this age, and the rest must be supplied by food—around 140mg.

Calcium-rich foods that are child- and smoothie-friendly include leafy greens (½ cup, 50mg to 100mg), homemade almond milk (½ cup, 47mg), yogurt (¼ cup, 110mg), oats (¼ cup, 11mg), calcium-enriched milks/dairy milk (½ cup, 150mg). Hence, a smoothie made with as little as a quarter cup of milk or yogurt for a baby is more than halfway to supplying the daily requirement for calcium from complementary foods. Toddlers who continue to be breastfed will need around 400mg from other sources, versus 500mg if they don't breastfeed. A smoothie including one cup of calcium-rich milk and half a cup of greens is 350mg to 400mg on its own.

It has been discussed in previous chapters that calcium is needed for healthy bones, teeth, and muscles, and vitamin D is needed to utilize calcium. According to the NHMRC in Australia, vitamin D requirements do not change from babies through adolescence at 5mcg (or 200IU) daily. For infants, 2.5mcg (100IU) is the amount considered necessary to prevent rickets in the absence of sunlight exposure. However, the Vitamin D Council in the United States suggests that babies need as much as 1000IU daily. Vitamin D can also be boosted via breast milk if Mother takes a high-dose supplement of vitamin D3 in the vicinity of 4000IU to 6000IU, which is significantly more than the 400IU in most supplements designed for pregnant and lactating women.

Vitamin D may be supplied in small degree by the addition of raw eggs to smoothies after the child is 1 year old, but this will not supply the amount needed. The best thing is to drink that smoothie in the sun!

Protein

Needed for growth, protein supplied by breast milk in the first 6 months is the right amount a baby needs, and based on the average intake of breast milk during this time, babies require around 10g of protein daily. This increases to 14g from 6 months and through to toddlerhood. With milk consumption reducing as complementary foods are introduced, it is expected such foods will provide half of this amount, or 7g. This is easily met via a serving of approximately a quarter cup of meat, cheese, or most nuts/seeds, one egg, one scant cup of cooked quinoa, one cup of dairy milk, or a half cup of cooked lentils. A cup of cooked greens will supply almost that amount (or the equivalent volume raw, given greens reduce and pack closely when cooked.) Some of these volumes are going to be too much for a baby and even for some toddlers, especially if choosing vegan options, as appetite often reduces as their growth rate decreases.

A well-planned vegetarian or vegan diet will supply enough protein provided a balance of grains, legumes, and nuts is eaten to ensure that all of the building blocks of protein and amino acids are consumed, plus the consumption of complete plant proteins. However, this may be difficult if you have a baby with a small appetite, a fussy toddler, and/or a child with food sensitivities to eggs, dairy, and/or nuts (which are rather common). As discussed previously, grains, nuts, and seeds lack lysine, and legumes lack methionine; however, chia, soy, and quinoa are complete proteins from the plant kingdom, which means they contain all eight essential amino acids. I don't recommend chia or soy for babies or toddlers, however—more on that later.

Smoothie-friendly protein sources for children: Raw eggs (for children over 1 year old), cooked quinoa, dairy milk, and yogurt all provide complete protein. For a toddler, one egg provides half their protein requirement for the day, as well as nuts and other seeds in the form of whole nuts/seeds, butters, or milks. The best options for protein additions to smoothies are almonds, cashews, and hemp and sunflower seeds. Pumpkin seeds have more protein than these but they have a stronger, less pleasant taste. Nuts and seeds will lack the amino acid lysine, so other sources of lysine should be consumed in the diet, which are generally from legumes or complete proteins. A source of lysine doesn't need to be in the same smoothie, but it's a good idea to include it as part of the diet somewhere else in the day. Peanuts are a legume, so the addition of peanut butter to a smoothie not only is delicious but also complements a smoothie with nuts in it, such as almond milk. More on the introduction of potentially allergenic foods like nuts will be discussed later in the chapter.

Vitamin A

Vitamin A needs increase by 40 percent in 7- to 12-month-olds from 250mcg to 430mcg, and this lowers to 300mcg for toddlers. The concentration available in breast milk remains the same at 310mcg per liter. About 500ml to 600ml is considered the average breast milk (or formula) intake by 7- to 12-month-olds, and so around 275mcg is needed from complementary foods for older babies, 150mcg for toddlers still being breastfed, and 300mcg if they are not. For more information on vitamin A, see Chapter 3, "Making Babies."

Smoothie-friendly vitamin A/beta-carotene sources for children: raw eggs (for children over 1 year old), carrots, pumpkin, sweet potato, spinach, kale, cantaloupe, mango, papaya, pineapples, passion fruit, apricots, peaches, nectarines, and kiwi

••

Premature Births

Assuming a mother isn't living in poverty and her baby was born to term, then vitamin A deficiency is unlikely, provided appropriate foods are supplied to the baby from 6 months. However, premature babies are not born with adequate liver stores of vitamin A, and this has a domino effect with the likelihood of deficiency throughout the first year of life. Subsequently, there is increased risk of eye, lung, and gastrointestinal diseases. Hence, it's extra important that attention is paid to supplying preemie babies enough vitamin A once solids are introduced.

With regard to preemies, similar issues with requiring supplementation and extra attention to diet exist with calcium, phosphorus, vitamin D, iron, zinc, copper, selenium, folate, DHA, and protein. Supplementation and the specific dietary needs of preemies are beyond the scope of this book, and prescriptions and advice should be given by the appropriate health professionals looking after these babies.

••

CONCERNS

To reiterate, the key reason why solids are introduced is for nutrition. The key nutrients above are the most important ones to provide babies from food sources other than breast milk or formula. Without them, babies risk stunted growth, inadequate brain development, eye disease, lowered immunity, and skeletal problems, some of which are irreversible, such as brain development. It should be noted that the demand for these nutrients isn't overnight when the baby reaches 6 months old; it is a gradual process that will vary according to the quality of stores the baby has. Moreover, breast milk or formula will gradually decrease as food intake increases, so the contribution of each source keeps changing and you should consider the recommended daily allowances for babies between 6 and 12 months as averages over this time.

It worries me when I hear of mothers choosing to feed their older babies only breast milk because they think "breast is best" or "breast is enough." After 6 months, breast milk plus food is better than breast milk (or formula) only. Another concern is the concept of "food before 1 is just for fun," which is something proponents of baby-led weaning (BLW) tend to favor. Personally, I love the concept of BLW and have used it, but not purely. Yes, food should be fun, but not "just for fun," because this approach can backfire, with babies potentially suffering deficiencies from not enough food intake, or not enough of the right foods. More on BLW and other methods of feeding will be discussed later in this chapter.

When to Introduce Solids

This topic should be quite straightforward, but it is far from it. Currently, the majority of relevant authorities around the world recommend that the introduction of solids be around 6 months, and that they should definitely not be introduced before 4 months. However, surveys worldwide show that it is very common for solids to begin between 4 and 6 months, and surprisingly, before 4 months.

There are many reasons for variation in the timing for introducing solids. Much of the confusion lies in the fact that there has been so much change in recommendations over the past century. In the early 1900s it was recommended to avoid solids except orange juice and cod liver oil until a baby was 12 months old. With the rise of the use of non-human milks and the promotion of prepackaged baby foods by the 1950s, breastfeeding rates had plummeted and solids were recommended to be introduced from 3 to 6 weeks and as early as 2 days old! In the 1970s the recommendation was from 4 months, in the 1980s it was between 3 and 4 months, and in the 1990s it was 4 to 6 months. Since 2001 the World Health Organization (WHO), and the majority of national organizations worldwide, recommend introduction of solids around 6 months.

Mothers naturally seek guidance from the mother figures in their lives, and if they started feeding solids to their children at 6 weeks or 3 months of age, they are likely to recommend the same to new mothers they know. Not everyone keeps up with guidelines from authorities such as the WHO or medical authorities of their country, such as the American Academy of Pediatrics (AAP), Department of Health (DOH) in the UK, or Australia's National Health and Medical Research Council (NHMRC). You would expect that doctors and nurses that deal with maternal and child health would know about these changes and disseminate the up-to-date information, but this is not always the case. And whether or not parents receive this information, they may choose to do it the way they think is right anyway. There is a lot to be said for instinct when it comes to parenting, but when it comes to feeding children, much of this "instinct" is misguided. Just like there are misconceptions about breast milk supply, as discussed in Chapter 5, "After the Baby Is Born," the same can be said for the introduction of solids.

Organizations that support the recommendation for the introduction for solids at or around 6 months include the following:

Global—The WHO, UNICEF, La Leche League, International Baby Food Action Network, International Confederation of Midwives, International Council of Nurses, International Pediatric Association, World Alliance for Breastfeeding Action, International Lactation Consultant Association, International Baby Food Action Network

USA—American Academy of Pediatrics (AAP), American College of Obstetrics and Gynecology, the American Academy of Family Physicians, Breastfeeding USA

Canada—Canadian Pediatric Society's Nutrition and Gastroenterology Committee, Dietitians of Canada, Breastfeeding Committee for Canada, Public Health Agency of Canada, Health Canada

Australia—National Health and Medical Research Council (NHMRC), Australian Breastfeeding Association, Nutrition Australia, Dietitians Association of Australia, the Royal Australian College of General Practitioners, the Royal Australian College of Physicians

New Zealand—Ministry of Health, Dietitians New Zealand

UK—Department of Health, National Health Service, British Dietetic Association

Europe—Karolinska Institute (Sweden), Institute for Child Health (Italy), European Commission (Public Health Directorate), Union of National European Pediatric Societies and Associations, European Association of Perinatal Medicine, European Federation of Nurses Associations, European Lactation Consultant Association, European Midwives Association, Federation of

European Nutrition Societies, European Society for Pediatric Gastroenterology, Hepatology, and Nutrition (ESPGHAN)

Organizations that support the 6-month introduction of solids have adopted the WHO guidelines. The WHO bases their recommendation on their systematic review findings of the available literature. Their findings suggest that:

> *exclusive breastfeeding of infants with only breast milk, and no other foods or liquids, for 6 months has several advantages over exclusive breastfeeding for 3 to 4 months followed by mixed breastfeeding. These advantages include a lower risk of gastrointestinal infection for the baby, more rapid maternal weight loss after birth, and delayed return of menstrual periods. No reduced risks of other infections or of allergic diseases have been demonstrated. No adverse effects on growth have been documented with exclusive breastfeeding for 6 months.*[1]

Organizations that support the recommendation for the introduction for solids between 4 and 6 months include:

The American Academy of Allergies Asthma and Immunology (AAAAI)

Australasian Society of Clinical Immunology and Allergy (ASICA)

European Food Safety Authority (EFSA)

STARTING TOO EARLY

While I personally believe we should make decisions regarding the introduction of food to our babies based on scientific evidence, it's still rather unclear whether it should be around 6 months

---

[1] http://www.who.int/mediacentre/news/statements/2011/breastfeeding_20110115/en

or 4 months! Much of the opinion surrounding the introduction from 4 months is based on allergies. Since the 1950s, allergic diseases have dramatically increased in the Western world. Australia, where I live, has one of the highest allergy rates in the world. Up to 40 percent of Australian children have evidence of allergic sensitization, which is similar to the United States. Many theories have been investigated including environmental factors such as exposure to allergens or toxins while in utero or while breastfeeding, the role of infections, antibiotic use in the first year, and use of probiotics—none of which has any conclusive evidence to base any recommendations on.

Similarly, there is still insufficient evidence to support when the "right time" to introduce solids is exactly. What is known, however, is that introduction before 4 months is absolutely NOT advised due to an increased risk of chronic diseases, such as diabetes, obesity, eczema, and celiac disease. A 2013 study by the CDC reported the results of a survey taken between 2005 and 2007 (when the guidelines were for introduction between 4 and 6 months). It was revealed that 40 percent of mothers were introducing solids *before* 4 months and over half of those did so upon medical advice, which is rather concerning. The most cited personal reasons were:

"My baby was old enough to begin eating solid food." Science tells us that before 4 months this is unwise.

"My baby seemed hungry a lot of the time." Babies' brains are very immature, and the reasons they get cranky and cry are many and varied and not always related to hunger. Babies also go through growth spurts, and around 3 months is a known period of extra growth that requires extra milk only.

"My baby wanted the food I ate or in other ways showed an interest in solid food." From 5 to 6 weeks of age, babies are increasingly interested in the world around them and this will include anything their parents do, including eating. They will also be interested in a dirty shoe put in front of them! From around 3 months, babies also begin exploring by putting anything and everything in their mouth—this does not mean they want or need to eat, it's simply learning about their world.

"I wanted to feed my baby something in addition to breast milk or formula." Sometimes motherhood can get a bit repetitive in the early days, but introducing solids early out of boredom or just "wanting to" isn't appropriate.

"It would help my baby sleep longer at night." Some parents claim that solids help their baby sleep, but there is no evidence to support this scientifically. There may also be other reasons babies sleep better at night and improvements in sleep are likely to be coincidental, particularly if this coincides with a developmental leap. Leaps are a term coined in the book *The Wonder Weeks* by Hetty van de Rijt and Frans Plooij. During a child's first 20 months, they go through 10 leaps, and during these leaps their learning and brain development is accelerated. During leaps, babies are fussier, cry more, and they often have regression of sleep quality, waking more times a night and it's harder to get to sleep. The first 4 leaps start at 5, 8, 12, and 15 weeks. Leap 3 is just 1 week starting at 12 weeks, so if the baby is fussing a lot at 3 months and is given solids and then settles, it is likely due to the leap ending, not from being given food. Leap 4 is a tough one and lasts 5 weeks, from week 15 to 19. This period between 4 and 5 months is frequently very unsettled for babies and is often misinterpreted as a time that solids are required to help settle them.

"I was worried that I was not producing enough milk." As discussed in the previous chapter, around 3 to 4 months, or earlier in some women, the breasts still produce ample milk, but they feel softer and babies become MUCH more efficient at suckling. Draining a breast in 3 to 5 minutes is not uncommon and is not a sign that a baby is disinterested in nursing, or that milk supply is dropping. If your baby is content after their feeds, and they are gaining weight, look healthy, and are generally active, then your milk supply is fine!

WHY YOU SHOULD WAIT

One reason given by supporters of waiting till 6 months to introduce solids is due to the gut being "open" prior to this. The gaps between cells in an immature gut are wider than a mature one, to allow large immune-protective proteins from breast milk through. This will of course allow other larger molecules through, too, so if solids are given before the gut "closes" around 6 months, this may introduce pathogens and proteins into the babies' bloodstream. This is one reason why exclusive breastfeeding is the most hygienic thing to do.

Those who support the earlier introduction of solids believe that there is potentially a critical window of opportunity to introduce potentially allergenic foods, to reduce the chances of allergies developing, and some research shows this to be between 4 and 6 months. These same supporters also emphasize the importance of maintaining breastfeeding during this period and healthy gut flora. Perhaps the open gut is a necessary part of this critical window? The thing is that at this point in time, we really don't know enough to be sure.

We do know not to introduce solid food before 4 months due to the risk of allergies and disease development, and that delaying solids is not good nutritionally (and possibly allergy-inducing too). Research is starting to support introduction of solids between 4 and 6 months, but the majority of guidelines worldwide say to introduce at or around 6 months. So what to do? Until guidelines are in the majority about introducing from 4 months, aiming for around 6 months is best practice.

Many parents decide to start solids at 4 months, and many doctors and nurses suggest this as well for no particular reason—just because you can doesn't mean you should. The fact is, many babies simply are not ready. Varying guidelines abound about establishing a child's "readiness" to start solids, and I recommend that you read any reliable resource about this topic.

SIGNS YOUR BABY IS READY FOR SOLIDS

Baby should be able to sit independently. Not many babies are sitting really well at 6 months, let alone at 4 months, and some normal babies are very late developers. A friend of mine's baby didn't sit well till nearly 1 year old, which would be far too late to start solids! A baby can be held on a parent's lap or supported in a high chair with cushions if needed. The most important part is that they are upright and have good head control (see next point).

Baby should have good head control. This is an absolute must as it's important for a baby to be able to accept food into the mouth, move it around in their mouth, and learn to chew and swallow, which is more advanced than the action for sucking in milk. Most babies have very good head control by 6 months and even 4 months, so this should not be an issue provided solids aren't introduced earlier than this.

Baby has lost its tongue-thrust reflex (TTR). This reflex is protective to a baby against choking as the tongue pushes food (or other objects) that are put in the mouth back out again. Trying to feed a baby with an active TTR is rather frustrating! Most babies lose this reflex around 6 months, some earlier and some later. My daughter didn't fully lose hers until she was about 7 months.

Baby is interested in watching adults eat and starts to grab for food. This is a tricky one. Certainly if your baby isn't interested that is pretty clear, but babies increasingly explore using their mouths from 3 months and are more and more interested in their environment from 5 to 6 weeks, so their interest in mealtimes may simply be interest in general and not an indication they want or need to start eating solids.

Baby shows an increased demand for milk feeds that is unrelated to illness, teething pain, a change in routine, or a growth spurt. This can be difficult to be sure about, as growth spurts tend to occur at 3, 4, and 6 months. The key thing is the demand is prolonged and not just for a few days or a week. In combination with the preceding three points, this is a very good indication your baby is ready to start solids. Increased demand is not typical of a large baby. Many smaller babies are very hungry babies and many large babies are perfectly happy on exclusive milk feeds till 6 months.

Baby is developing pincer grip. True pincer grip, picking up small items between the tips of the thumb and index finger, won't happen until 9 to 11 months but preparing for this with more of a crude scooping action is around 7 to 8 months. Hence, waiting for this would delay solids. It is very important but not needed to begin eating.

Baby opens mouth when offered food from a spoon. This is fairly obvious as being necessary to begin solids. If their mouth stays shut, no food will go in! If you've decided to use purely baby-led weaning (more on this later in the chapter), then no spoons are offered; rather, it's the baby starting finger foods from day 1, and there will still need to be a willingness to open their mouth to accept the finger food being offered.

As a medical doctor and mum of three, I have had the benefit of a varied experience with my children and their readiness for solids. With my eldest, she was always a very hungry baby. Around 4 months she started breastfeeding more frequently throughout the day—every 1 to 2 hours all day and demanding frequent night feeds again. I didn't actually think it was hunger, but my mother did. I was nervous because "the baby books" at that time said wait till 6 months. I resisted for another week or so, but she was clearly not sick, wasn't teething, and I just couldn't keep up with the demand. When I offered her some solids off a spoon, she ate a whole bowlful with gusto and was on three meals a day in less than a week!

My second wasn't even remotely interested before 6 months. We attempted a couple of times given my eldest had started so early, but it was clear she wasn't interested—she didn't know what to do with the food in her mouth, and she hadn't had any signs of an increased need for breast milk. Not long after 6 months I noticed that same pattern of feeding more frequently, and she used to watch us eat like a hawk—once she started she wasn't quite as quick as her sister but still eating lots within a couple of weeks.

By the time our third child came along we were quite relaxed. She was always very interested in her sisters, and around 5 months she used to intently watch them eat and even seemed a bit upset when they were eating and she wasn't. Then one of them gave her some banana and we were off! —Megan

IN SUMMARY

Your baby should begin solids around 6 months when showing signs of readiness, including having good head control, loss of tongue-thrust reflex, and a willingness to take food into the mouth. Start offering food around 5 to 5½ months to test for readiness, and if not interested or not ready, then try again a week later. What to offer will be discussed in the next sections. It is acceptable to begin to introduce solids with signs of readiness from 4 months if there is a prolonged increased demand for feeds as discussed above. Don't introduce solids before 4 months (17 weeks) and avoid delaying beyond 7 months. Do not introduce solids at 4 months (or earlier) just because your baby is big or small, because they wake overnight, or because they cry a lot—this includes avoiding putting cereal in a baby's bottle.

DELAYING FOODS

With the increasing incidence of allergies in recent decades, it was previously thought that delaying potentially allergenic foods would prevent the onset of allergies. Common guidelines included avoiding eggs till 2 years old and no peanuts or tree nuts or fish till 3 years old. Unfortunately, allergies kept climbing, and it is possible that guidelines to delay these foods have played a part in this. Given this, it is now recommended that *nothing be delayed* for allergy reasons, including gluten, dairy, eggs, tree nuts, peanuts, and fish.

Depending on your source, particularly books and websites, it is still common to see recommendations to delay foods, including those mentioned above, as well as legumes (especially red kidney beans), meat, gluten, dairy, citrus, strawberries, kiwi, pineapple, leafy greens, onions, and garlic. Some resources provide timetables of what to introduce and when according to age, with different fruit and veg over three to four different time frames. Seriously, it's hard enough coordinating when in the day to try and feed your baby in those first few months, let alone being so restricted with what foods to offer!

ONE FOOD AT A TIME?

In addition to current evidence not supporting the delay of any food for allergy reasons, beyond 6 months it is also not necessary to introduce one food type at a time. However, those that support the introduction of solids between 4 and 6 months do recommend introducing one food at a time and watching for any reactions. You can't introduce a lot of variety in a short time anyway, and as you settle in to your staples, you will add in new foods between 6 and 12 months and even beyond. You will notice if something has a reaction, such as adding some strawberries to a banana smoothie, when you know that banana smoothies have been fine; if baby's butt gets a bit red the next day when that meal comes out as poo, or a bit of a rash forms around the baby's mouth, then perhaps the strawberries are a bit irritating. You can then try it again in a few weeks. Some babies' react to certain fruits like this and others don't. There is no need to avoid it "just in case." Try it and see what happens. My daughter has diagnosed sensitivities to cashews, almonds, wheat, and eggs, but she is fine with all fruits and vegetables including garlic and onions.

A Note about Rice Cereal

Standard advice is to begin foods with baby rice cereal: mix up a little in water or milk starting with 1 to 2 teaspoons, which makes it quite runny at first, but you gradually mix it up thicker. Once the baby can manage plain cereal, then mixing it with fruit or veggie purees is often suggested. Commercial baby rice cereals are essentially devoid of nutrition apart from the fact they are fortified with iron—which we know older babies need from food. My maternal child health nurse suggested using it initially as it was easy to mix up 1 to 2 teaspoons at a time versus making a fruit puree that would supply a lot more than 2 teaspoons. You could say it's easy, though another view is that it's lazy. That may sound harsh, but yes, making a homemade puree is more effort initially; however, then you have multiple servings available to freeze. Plus, a homemade puree is *real* food that is nutritious, as opposed to highly processed cereal that must be fortified because it is so lacking in nutrients. My nurse did emphasize that it's important to move on to real foods fairly quickly once babies get the hang of eating off a spoon. Even though I chose not to use cereal at all, I was pleased she was giving out this advice, although I still see many mothers using rice cereals in purees month after month, and not quickly moving on to lumpier foods and finger foods (more on that later in the chapter).

Rice cereals are also recommended because they are highly unlikely to provoke an allergic reaction. Many parents use rice cereals happily and don't see what the fuss is all about with those that are against them. I won't tell you not to use them as they aren't exactly poisonous, and it's your choice how to feed your children, but I am not a fan and think there are much better alternatives to babies' first foods. Many experts agree that providing rice cereal to babies' is akin to giving them spoonfuls of sugar—we would never literally do such a thing, but starchy carbohydrates such as rice cereal turn quite rapidly into sugar in the body. This is why many adults avoid "carbs" and more and more people are quitting sugar, as they learn how harmful sugar is to the human body—obesity, diabetes, and heart disease are just a few serious conditions that high sugar consumption contributes to, not to mention mental health conditions, such as anxiety, and digestive disorders, such as colitis and Crohns.

It is very common to see children from an early age get hooked on grain foods. The pattern of cereal for breakfast, a sandwich for lunch, pasta for dinner, and grain-based snacks in between do not do children any favors when it comes to risk of future type 2 diabetes and struggles with weight and behavior. This diet is not helped when three servings of whole grains daily are advised for toddlers for reasons of supplying fiber. I am not suggesting no grains should be consumed, but less of them and greater variety is required. As adults we should ideally avoid eating the same thing over and over, which is quite typical of many people's breakfasts. Even the same smoothie every day is not wise, especially if it has leafy greens in it (see "Mix Up Your Greens" on page 3 about the importance of rotating greens). There is a lot of compelling reading in publications such as Dr. David Perlmutter's *Grain Brain* and *Gut and Psychology Syndrome* by Dr. Natasha Campbell-McBride, discussing the science behind the danger of grains and sugar—including inflammation of the brain, addiction to grains from the opioid-type substances they contain, and candida overgrowth in the gut. With regard to babies and toddlers, flooding the diet with grains is bad news. Grain foods are delicious, easy to eat, and addictive. What may start as an innocent piece of bread for an infant turns into daily bread, daily cereal, daily crackers, and daily pasta or rice, and with so much grain (and usually it is all wheat, which contains gluten) there is less of the good stuff, such as fruit, veggies, and good fat and protein sources. Feeding you baby or toddler a smoothie for breakfast or lunch is a great start to substituting what may already be a multiple times a day grain habit, or to helping prevent this from happening. In addition, smoothies are a great source of fiber!

••

The Best Smoothies for Babies and Toddlers

We have discussed already that no foods are off limits for allergy-prevention reasons and that no particular order is necessary to introduce foods to babies. If introducing food before 6 months, my recommendation is to wait till after 6 months to introduce smoothies, given they generally have multiple ingredients and you don't want to risk filling up a baby on a smoothie that may displace a milk feed—no matter how fancy your smoothie combo is it will never be as nutritious and calorie dense as breast milk or formula. One risk of introducing solids before 6 months is the risk of baby having less milk. Under 6 months, solids should be in addition to the same quantity of milk they were drinking. It's after 6 months that milk feeds gradually reduce as solids increase.

I suggest when creating your own smoothies or following my recipes for younger babies that the ingredients used have been eaten before without issue, or just one ingredient is new, for example, a smoothie with bananas, almond milk, and spinach, when they have eaten almonds and banana previously.

For children under 1 year old, ingredients to *not* put in smoothies include raw eggs (and never if not the very best quality) and honey due to risk (albeit a very tiny risk) of botulism contamination, which younger systems can't destroy. Foods like whole nuts, whole grapes, raw carrot chunks, etc., which are choking hazards for young children, should also be avoided generally.

Smoothies for babies and toddlers are no different from adult smoothies in that they are a combination of non-liquid and liquid foods blended together. The non-liquid ingredients may be fruits, vegetables, leafy greens, nuts, seeds, and grains. The liquid ingredients may be water, coconut water, juice, or milk.

FRUITS

Fruits that are easily mashed and eaten raw such as banana, avocado, mango, papaya, watermelon, blueberries, and ripe and soft pears and stone fruit are great for baby smoothies. Fruits that tend to be cooked for baby purees, such as apples, firm pears, and firm stone fruits, are also great additions in a cooked (and cooled) form. Sweeteners should be minimized in baby and toddler food, including smoothies. Instead, use sweet fruit like bananas, ripe pears, mangoes, and melons, or use iron-rich dried fruit in moderation, such as raisons, prunes, dates, and apricots. Soak dried fruit overnight to rehydrate, making them easier to blend. Fruits are a great source of vitamins (especially vitamin C), antioxidants (including beta-carotene, the precursor to vitamin A), and fiber. Fiber from fruits is more of the soluble type, which means it dissolves in the gut and helps soften and form stools. This is in contrast to insoluble fiber, which breaks down into smaller pieces and passes through the digestive tract, acting like a broom to keep things moving and grooving! Too little fiber and fluids will lead to constipation, whereas the opposite can lead to loose stools. When solids are introduced there needs to be a balance of some but not too much fiber. Many are familiar with constipation from not enough fiber, but too much can also lead to uncomfortable tummies with gas and bloating, and if food passes too quickly through the digestive tract, it may adversely affect nutrient absorption. Blueberries and pears are particularly good sources of smoothie-friendly soluble fiber to use if your little one is a bit constipated. My daughter loves eating blueberries; she gets to practice her pincer grip and just devours them. I am sure she would eat them for every meal, but she most certainly does "blueberry poos" less than 24 hours later, so I limit them to a couple of times a week, whether whole or in a smoothie.

Some experts recommend limiting fruit to babies, as it may give them a sweet tooth, and to focus on veggies instead, but fruit is a good source of calories and is easy and convenient to give babies and toddlers. Breast milk is also very sweet; try it if you haven't before! Babies will have a sweet tooth already for lack of a better word, and once introducing solids it's time to expand on their palate to include savory foods. Sure, don't feed you baby just fruit, but fruit is natural, delicious, and far better than processed or baked goods that contain sugar.

VEGETABLES AND LEAFY GREENS

Many kids, particularly as they enter the toddler years, struggle with veggie consumption. According to my survey, the most common feeding problems mothers reported were with "some vegetables" followed by "anything new," "greens," "most vegetables," "some fruits," and lastly "most fruits." There are many reasons why kids have aversions to vegetables, particularly non-starchy ones, but one of them is that they can fill up small tummies quickly without providing many calories. Babies grow rapidly in their first 3 to 6 months, with growth rate declining slowly and definitely slower by 1 year of age, and with this can come a smaller appetite. It is not uncommon for older babies to eat more than toddlers. Veggies are important and a great source of vitamins, minerals, antioxidants, and fiber, but kids may find them unappealing because they are not overly satisfying. Rather, they would prefer starchy foods for energy, and this is where favoring grain foods and potatoes tends to take off. Still, persist with a variety of veggies in the diet as a whole and don't stress about veg not being eaten in significant quantities, but try making them tempting and more nutritious by serving them with fat, such as steamed broccoli dipped in lots of good-quality butter or coconut oil. Remember that fat is needed to help absorb minerals and the fat-soluble vitamins A, E, D, and K, so it's important to add some fat to your smoothie as well.

Many parents find they need to hide veggies in their cooking. About 43 percent of mothers in my survey reported hiding veggies finely grated in things like pasta sauces, and 26 percent used smoothies in a similar way. Most people identify smoothies as being a fruit-based drink, but veggies can play a role too: An inch of raw or cooked carrot or beet can easily be snuck into a smoothie However, you need a good-quality, high-speed blender to break raw vegetables down well, otherwise the mouthfeel won't be pleasant. Beets create a gorgeous pink color that is very attractive to kids, and they are very nutritious, particularly raw. Moreover, root veg like beets and carrots are sweet and combine well with fruit, which is useful for creating a variety of smoothie recipes.

Vegetable juices used as the liquid base are also an option, which eliminates potentially excessive fiber in the smoothie compared to using whole pieces of veg, but the nutrition from the veg is still there. Juices consumed on their own are not recommended for kids for reasons of dental hygiene, but when used in a smoothie it is not an issue. The smoothie can be consumed as a meal or snack and the mouth rinsed afterward or teeth brushed, as opposed to grazing over the smoothie for hours, which will leave sugars in the mouth that may affect dental health. A smoothie also contains fiber, which slows down the metabolism of sugar in the digestive tract, to avoid highs and lows of blood sugar, which in kids can affect behavior, including eating behaviors—more on that later in the chapter. One issue with using juices, particularly if making them yourself (which is ideal to avoid consuming heat-treated juices, preservatives, etc.) is that it means another step and appliance in the smoothie-making process, which can create inconvenience, something that smoothies alone tend to avoid.

Depending on your source, some say raw veggies are too hard on the digestion of infants and should be cooked, and others say it's fine. The beauty of making smoothies, however, is that the blending process ruptures the cell membranes of the plant foods used, releasing nutrients that otherwise can have a hard time being released by chewing raw veg alone. Cooking also breaks down cell membranes, but it can also denature protein and destroy some nutrients, such as vitamin C and antioxidant pigments in beets. However, cooking can also enhance nutrient availability in veggies, reducing the goitrogenic effect of brassicas and to a lesser degree spinach, which is better for iodine absorption. Hence, it is an option to steam greens and sweet root veg (carrot, beet, sweet potato, pumpkin) to add to smoothies, which also makes them easier to blend and taste sweeter. I would not recommend raw sweet potato or pumpkin, however. My recipes do not contain cooked greens; however, this is certainly possible.

NUTS AND SEEDS

A great source of minerals such as calcium, zinc, magnesium, and selenium, as well as vitamin E, good fats, and protein, nuts and seeds are a great way of adding calories and nutrition to a smoothie. They are also great for adding creaminess, which is something that in combination with sweetness is attractive to many smoothie-drinking kiddies.

Nuts and seeds, however, can be a source of allergies and sensitivities in some children, particularly peanuts (actually a legume), almonds, cashews, and sesame seeds. As discussed, delaying the introduction of nuts and seeds is not advised, even if a parent has sensitivities or allergies themselves. It is wise, however, to introduce individual nuts and seeds one at a time and watch for any problems, such as rash around the mouth, eczema, abdominal pain, vomiting, change in bowel habit, red bottom, etc. They may be included in a meal with other foods, but try only one at a time and if there is not any problem, then you can include them in smoothies.

If confident about the addition of new nuts and seeds, there are many ways to add them to a smoothie. A nut milk such as almond milk can be used as the liquid base, and whole nuts or nut butter can also be added. Other tasty and healthy options for children include hemp and sunflower seeds, cashews, and macadamias. If time allows and you remember, soaking the nuts or seeds overnight in filtered water and draining/rinsing them before use adds to their digestibility and nutrient availability. Exceptions are hemp seeds, which are phytate-free and don't require pre-soaking.

Chia Seeds

Chia seeds have become very trendy in recent years and recipes for infants that include them are popular, but I do not recommend these for babies and toddlers. Chia is promoted as a great source of omega-3 fats, calcium, magnesium, iron, soluble fiber, and protein. On the surface it sounds like the perfect baby food! But let's break it down. Chia is replete with omega-3s, but this is omega-3 ALA. DHA is the omega-3 fat that is most important for infants, especially for the first 2 years, being essential for their brain and nervous system development. The conversion of ALA to DHA is minimal, and hence it's better to get DHA into your baby's diet via breast milk (or formula with DHA), DHA supplements for kids, and/or eating seafood. Chia also contains phytates that bind to minerals such as the ones chia contains; the bound minerals are then expelled from the body in its waste products. However, when soaked, chia forms a gel, hanging onto the soak water, which can't be rinsed away and hence the phytates stay put. Therefore, the mineral benefits of chia are debatable.

Fiber, as discussed already, is really important for babies who can be prone to constipation; however, too much can be a problem too. Chia's fiber can have quite a powerful laxative effect in small quantities in adults, let alone kids, and if the chia seeds are not consumed pre-soaked, they will soak up 10-plus times their size in water in the gut, which can slow things down, may cause discomfort, and will reduce fluid absorption into the bloodstream. Whether they are consumed unsoaked or pre-soaked, they still end up swollen in the gut, which is filling. However, we don't want to fill up young kids on low-calorie foods. They need nutritious food that will supply calories for energy and weight gain. The filling effect of chia, often consumed in the form of a chia pudding or added to smoothies or cereal, can be a great strategy for adults who are trying to lose weight. For kids it can reduce appetite and create what seems to be a "fussy child," but they are simply not hungry because they are full.

Lastly, in 2 tablespoons (or 20g) of chia there is 3.4g of protein and this is an adult serving. A child's serving of 1 teaspoon has less than 1g of protein, which is not a significant contribution to the 14g required daily by babies and toddlers from 6 months of age. Therefore, my recipes for babies and toddlers won't include chia seeds, unlike some of my adult smoothie recipes. If you disagree with me and wish to use them anyway, they will thicken up a smoothie, so bear that in mind with mastering the right consistency.

••

GRAINS

As discussed in Chapter 1 "The Art and Science of Making Smoothies," oats, quinoa, and millet feature in my smoothie recipes, including those for infants. I list all of these as cooked in this chapter, which omits raw oats as an option. This is because cooked oats will be digested more easily than raw, and if cooked as a porridge, they blend into a smoothie better so that the end result is lovely and smooth. Raw oats can leave a gritty mouthfeel that toddlers in particular won't be fond of. If you choose to feed your baby or toddler the grain-based smoothies regularly, I highly recommend freezing half-cup portions of the cooked grain so you can thaw them overnight in the fridge the day before you wish to use them.

FATS

I admit, I am guilty of banging on about good fats—but they are very, very important! Please refer back to Chapter 2, "Fabulous Fats," as a reminder if needed. In summary, here are the highlights.

About 97 percent of the human body's fat is saturated and monounsaturated, and 3 percent is polyunsaturated fat, half of which is omega-3. The most important omega-3 fats for infants are DHA, which is essential for brain, eye, and nervous system development, including its positive effects on mood and sleep. DHA represents 97 percent of all omega-3 fats in the brain, and 93 percent in the retina in the eye. The importance of DHA to the central nervous system extends from pregnancy and into the second year of a child's life. DHA is not a fat easily included in smoothie recipes unless it includes using expressed breast milk or formula that contains DHA. Otherwise DHA needs to come from these milk sources generally, seafood in the diet, and/or DHA supplementation. As discussed in Chapter 5, "After the Baby Is Born," the total fat in breast milk remains unchanged irrespective of diet; however, maternal DHA consumption influences the amount of DHA in breast milk. While lactating, women are recommended to supplement with at least 200mg to 300mg (and up to 1000mg according to other sources) in addition to a diet containing DHA-rich foods, namely seafood. Recommendations for DHA supplementation to infants is variable, but assuming the mother is able to supply sufficient DHA via breast milk then breastfed babies shouldn't need it, at least not until milk feeds reduce between 9 and 12 months. Often toddlers aged 1 to 2 years old eat less than when they were older babies and may not eat much, if any, seafood; hence, adding a daily DHA supplement in liquid form is a wise idea. If formula feeding, not all formulations contain DHA, so it's best to seek one out that does.

DHA is not the only important fat of course. Infants, children, and adults need to consume omega-3 and -6 in the correct ratio (1:1 to 1:3, not just by consuming sources of omega-3, but minimizing consumption of omega-6 from vegetable oils). Saturated fats, monounsaturated fats, and cholesterol are also very important. These are the fabulous fats that we can get into our smoothies to help with healthy cell function, to build hormones, and to absorb minerals and fat-soluble vitamins.

Smoothie-friendly fats for children: Coconut (milk, cream, and fresh soft flesh), avocado, macadamias, hemp, and walnuts. Still nutritious, but not as useful when it comes to fats, are other nuts and seeds such as cashews, almonds, and pecans, and sunflower and pumpkin seeds. Raw eggs (for the yolks) are not recommended for babies but can be introduced after the child is 1 year old, as long as the eggs are fresh and hygienic (see "Fats in Smoothies" on page 21).

WATER

We need water for hydration, detoxification, and elimination. The majority of our bodies are made up of water. As adults we need around 2 liters/8 cups of water daily, and toddlers need 1.3 liters/5 to 6 cups. This will include water that is contained in solids and in milk. Young babies do not need water in addition to breast milk or formula. Older babies are encouraged to take sips of water to get used to the taste and habit, but don't need a lot as they are still drinking breast milk or formula. Once babies become toddlers around 12 months, they will drink less milk and more water. The more active they are, the more water they will need, and water will gradually increase from sips as an older baby to 3 to 4 cups daily as an active toddler (this is taking into account fluid in foods plus the suggested 1 to 2 cups of milk for a toddler). Water or other fluids that go into a smoothie are of course part of what hydrates an older baby or toddler.

COCONUT WATER

In the center of fresh drinking coconuts is the delicious and delicately sweet water, which can be used interchangeably with plain water in a smoothie. As discussed on page 43, coconut water contains mineral electrolytes, such as calcium, magnesium, potassium, manganese, and sodium. It also contains vitamin C, and vitamins B2 and B6. It is sweetened by a low level of naturally occurring sugars (with a higher glucose:fructose ratio) and is very low in fat. Coconut water is wonderful to use in smoothies as it has a lovely flavor that isn't overpowering, is sweeter than water or milk, but not as sweet and sugary as many juices. This quality lends itself beautifully to smoothies for children who generally prefer a sweeter smoothie. A sweet liquid base to a smoothie is useful when adding nutritious fruits that aren't super sweet, such as berries, or when adding greens or cacao that are naturally bitter. Coconut water used as the sweetener will be a healthier choice than adding concentrated sweeteners such as syrups.

As discussed on page 45, you can open your own drinking coconuts and use the water fresh. Most coconuts supply 1 to 2 cups of liquid depending on the size of the coconut. Go for Thai coconuts, as they tend to taste the nicest. Alternatively, you can buy packaged coconut water, but go for the varieties that are 100 percent coconut water only.

JUICE

Juices may also be used as a part, or the entire liquid base, of a smoothie. Reasons to use juice over water or milk are for variety of flavor, color, and/or nutritional benefits. The use of root vegetable juices such as carrot or beet can provide a gorgeous hit of color, and anyone who has had a toddler to feed knows that something as simple as the color of a food, drink, cup, or plate can be very, very, very important! Beets and carrots are also naturally sweet and are chock-full of nutritious antioxidant pigments including beta-carotene, the precursor to vitamin A. You can put small pieces of raw or steamed carrot or beet into a smoothie, but if you want more nutrients in a smoothie without all the fiber, which can be very filling and heavy, then the juice is the way to go. Other juice options are apple or orange, which are very sweet and suit smoothies with tart berries or when introducing green smoothies. Non-sweet juices such as cucumber can be used too, which will be similar to using water but a little more nutritious, adding a little vitamin C, potassium, and magnesium. Be sure to use non-bitter cucumbers such as English or Persian varieties.

Juices are generally not recommended for children and especially older babies and toddlers for reasons of dental health, with concerns that the sugars in the juice sit on the teeth and contribute to decay. This is mostly of concern when they are sipped between meals; the same could be said for any sweet drink, including a smoothie. So whether it be a juice, a smoothie containing juice, or a smoothie not containing juice, don't have your child sip it slowly over hours. After it's drunk, have your child brush their teeth or at least rinse their mouth with water.

The other concern with kids drinking sweet fruit juices is that it is a big hit of sugar—often as much as in a soda (albeit more nutritious)—and unopposed by the presence of fiber. The benefit of a smoothie or smoothie-containing juice over a plain juice is that the former has fiber (assuming there is fruit, veg, and/or greens in the smoothie). Fiber slows the movement of glucose from food or drink into the bloodstream via the intestines. Rapid movement of glucose spikes blood sugar, which in kids and adults can affect mood and behavior. A child who is hyperactive on a sugar rush followed by a crash when blood sugar falls again is not a fun child to deal with. Therefore, avoid your child drinking plain juice between meals, and instead give fresh juice occasionally as part of a fiber-rich meal or in a smoothie.

If providing juices to your little ones, it is preferable that they are freshly squeezed by hand or in a juicer. For a start, they taste a million times better than anything in a bottle or carton. Commercial juices will also be heat treated to give them a shelf life. Heating destroys flavor in juices, as well as nutrients, especially vitamin C, and at high temperatures, folate. If you look at juice packets, frequently you will see vitamin C/ascorbic acid added back in. This will be synthetic vitamin C. It's much better to consume naturally occurring vitamin C from freshly squeezed juice! The disadvantage of making your own juice is inconvenience—compared to a smoothie that is very simple and quick, juicing is usually messy and time consuming. If going to the effort to make juice, make extra and use it in smoothies 2 to 3 days in a row, or freeze excess juice in ice block molds to use another day, either as ice or thawed out.

MILK

Looking at milk from a culinary perspective, there are many options—dairy milk; coconut milk; nut milks such as almond, macadamia, or cashew; seed milks such as hemp or sunflower; grain milks such as oat or rice; or soy milk from a legume. There is of course the option of formula or breast milk for baby and toddler smoothies, too. All milks will add creaminess to a smoothie that water or juice doesn't. It is a creaminess that generally isn't thick or potentially heavy, such as the creaminess from adding whole nuts, nut butters, avocado, or coconut flesh/cream. Coconut milk can still be quite rich depending on the source. Kids often prefer a smoothie that is somewhat creamy, so a milk base is ideal. Rice milk will provide the least creamy option and is a little sweet, as it is higher in carbohydrate. Breast milk or formula will be the sweetest.

Milk, depending on the variety, will also provide nutritional benefits. As discussed earlier, fluid requirements for active toddlers are 1.3 liters per day, inclusive of water, milk, juice, and food. Recommendations for toddler milk requirements are 350ml to 500ml per day to supply protein and calcium in particular. This recommendation is based on continuing to receive breast milk or cow's milk, with no more than 500ml of daily cow's milk because its high calcium content can interfere with iron absorption. This is one reason why breast milk is higher in calcium and low in iron.

Cow's milk, or any milk, does not *have* to be supplied to a toddler provided that adequate fluids, protein, and calcium are supplied elsewhere in the diet. If cow's milk isn't tolerated by your toddler, or you choose not to feed cow's milk to your child, then calcium-enriched soy milk or almond milk is usually suggested— both being a source of both protein and calcium. If your child can't have almonds or soy, then careful attention needs to be paid to your child getting nutrients that cow's milk and dairy products can provide simply and easily. I am in such a situation; however, my daughter does tolerate natural yogurt high in probiotic cultures and I continue to breastfeed. Soy milk however, should be used with caution, due to its very high phytoestrogen content. Soy is known to disrupt hormones in adults and of course children's systems are smaller and less developed, potentially creating more significant hormonal issues—at the extreme it can be early maturation of sexual organs.

Nut and seed milks are simple to make at home. Please refer to my recipe on page 12.

Recipes are also readily available online for homemade rice and coconut milks. If you are like me, however, and find that there is much less time to make everything from scratch when you have a young child, then using commercially made milk is otherwise suitable. Please do choose the best quality milks. Many non-dairy types of milk are available in 1-liter tetra packs, which makes storing them at home in your pantry very easy. Some, however, are full of unnecessary ingredients like gums, added sugars, and oils, so be an ingredient detective. Also try to choose organic options, which will guarantee they do not contain GMOs.

If your child is having formula, then that can be included in a smoothie, as can expressed breast milk. Even though many toddlers continue to drink formula after they turn 1, it is not necessary, as regular milk (namely cow's or almond) and food will provide the nutrition they need, and as already discussed, milk itself isn't compulsory. If you are breastfeeding and don't usually pump, I don't suggest you pump for the purpose of supplying smoothie milk, but if you have an excess of milk from pumping, either fresh or stored in the freezer, by all means use it in your child's smoothie—better this than it go to waste. Bear in mind if you use thawed milk, you can't freeze the smoothie it goes into in the event you have excess and hope to reserve it for later consumption—it will need to be drunk or thrown out. Breast milk and formula are both quite sweet so take that into account with other ingredients. For example, breast milk and ripe bananas will be sickly sweet, but breast milk and strawberries or blueberries would be fabulous!

OTHER INGREDIENTS

Frequently, "grown up" smoothies contain additional ingredients in smaller quantities, such as superfood powders; raw cacao; spices like cinnamon, cardamom, and ginger; protein powders; probiotics; or green powders. For the most part, I recommend keeping smoothies for infants pretty simple, and sticking to whole foods rather than powdered food options. Use real leafy greens over green powders and whole protein sources over protein powders—kids need protein to grow, but you don't want to overload them with it either. Spices are likely to be too strong in flavor for little ones, the exception being cinnamon, which is mild, and given its great for blood sugar balance, it may be useful for improving behavior by assisting with prevention of highs and lows with blood sugar imbalances. Raw cacao (or cocoa) is the bitter base of chocolate. It contains PEA (phenethylamine), which is a natural "feel good" chemical, and it is a good source of iron and magnesium; however, it also contains a small amount of caffeine and much greater quantities of theobromine, which is a stimulant similar to caffeine. My personal opinion is that cacao is best left out of baby and toddler diets because of its stimulating properties—we don't give young kids tea or coffee for this reason, so logic dictates cacao should stay out too. I know some parents who give their toddlers smoothies with cacao, but they use small amounts such as 1 to 2 flat teaspoons for a liter smoothie. My recommendation is that if you do choose to give your toddler cacao, don't supply it as part of a meal close to a nap time, use it with older rather than younger toddlers, keep amounts small, and if you think it makes them hyperactive, then best not to give it to them.

How to Introduce Solids

In addition to the confusion of when to introduce solids is the "how do you do it" part! Traditional and mainstream advice is to spoon-feed babies, beginning with 1 to 2 teaspoons of pureed fruit or root vegetable or rice cereal mixed with water or breast milk/formula. Then gradually increase the volume of puree, and gradually make the purees less smooth so your baby gets used to texture. Around 8 to 9 months, babies develop pincer grip and it's recommended that your baby begins feeding themselves with some finger foods, such as pieces of steamed veg, soft fruits, pieces of bread, etc. This will transition into eating family foods around age 1 while also learning to self-feed with eating utensils.

An alternative method of feeding is called baby-led weaning (BLW). The "weaning" part of this equation refers to the introduction of food, not the cessation of breastfeeding. The theory of BLW was developed by a UK midwife called Gill Rapley as part of her master's degree on babies' developmental readiness for solids. In her book of the same name, she explains that baby-led weaning is all about babies feeding themselves from the start—the start being around 6 months. At this age babies are well and truly picking up items and putting them to and in their mouth, so this skill can be used for feeding—it doesn't require pincer grip. Around 6 months, babies have a sensitive gag reflex, which is protective to choking. The stimulus for the gag reflex is further forward in the mouth at this age and if finger foods (or toys or anything else for that matter) are projected at or beyond this point, they gag. Understanding the difference between gagging and choking is very important, as gagging is no reason to jump into first-aid measures.

Advantages of BLW includes assisting hand-eye coordination, chewing skills (still effective even with just gums), bringing forward the sharing of family meals, and most importantly your baby leads the way, eating at a pace that suits them and stopping when full. Spoon-feeding has a tendency to result in overfeeding babies, as parents often sneak spoons of food in "to finish the bowl." BLW is touted as resulting in children that are less fussy eaters, thanks partly to the earlier introduction of textured foods.

Disadvantages of BLW include the potential delay of adequate amounts and varieties of solids, particularly if a baby doesn't take to it quickly. As discussed earlier, protein, calcium, vitamin A, iron, and zinc are of particular importance to a baby's diet after 6 months, as the amount they can get from breast milk or formula is limited compared to their needs to develop. Many babies take to BLW well and by 7 months are eating (chewing/swallowing) at least 2 to 3 tablespoons of food. However, some babies, like mine, take to it too slowly.

I loved the idea of BLW and wanted to do it purely, but after 5 to 6 weeks of trying, nothing much was happening. My daughter was happy to pick food up and put it in her mouth but most food just fell back out again—probably because it took till around 7 months for her tongue-thrust reflex to go. Munching on cucumber sticks was lovely on her gums, but a little cucumber flesh and watermelon wasn't going to cut it nutritionally. So I ended up doing a combined approach: I introduced some purees on spoons and persisted with finger foods, too. She thought I was mad by suddenly offering a spoon of glop after what she had been attempting, but after a week she had the hang of it and was actually swallowing food, and then her poo changed to let me know it! Before too long she didn't want to be spoon-fed and clearly wanted to feed herself, so I put blobs of thick or lumpy purees on her high-chair tray and pre-loaded spoons plus finger foods, which she was getting the hang of.

Introducing Smoothies

Your chosen method of introducing solids will dictate how you go about feeding your baby smoothies. If you are happy to start with spoon-feeding, then that makes it quite easy. If you want to purely do BLW, then it's a little trickier. The following methods are all possibilities for introducing smoothies—try them and see what works for you.

If starting early with smoothies then you will likely only give a small amount, so it's most logical to make a smoothie to share—be it with another child or yourself, keeping it simple and using appropriate ingredients for your baby—just try a single fruit and milk, water, or coconut water. You can also blend up a basic combo, and take some out and then add more into it for you. (I offer specific suggestions in the following recipe section.) When you are confident that your baby is okay with a variety of foods, then as long as the smoothie doesn't contain raw eggs or honey, sharing a smoothie with more ingredients in it is fine. When your older baby or toddler can handle a much larger volume, then making their own smoothie becomes more practical (and after your child is 1 year old, it may include raw eggs and honey). However, many mothers make the same smoothie and share it with their kids anyway, and according to my survey, this figure was almost 50 percent.

SPOON-FEED

Just like you would feed a baby a spoon of puree, you can feed them a spoon of smoothie. Given a smoothie will be runnier than a puree, a deeper spoon will work best as it will hold a better volume. Thick foods and purees can sit above the level of a spoon, but a smoothie won't. In terms of how may teaspoons to offer, be guided by your baby—if they are opening their mouth wanting more, then offer more. Don't force or sneak spoons of smoothie in. If they don't want it, they don't want it. They may not like the taste or they are full. If you force things, you will likely see that smoothie back up again! Spoon-feeding is appropriate for a younger baby, but if you are introducing smoothies to an older baby or toddler, then try one of the other methods discussed below. Older babies and toddlers are hopefully not being spoon-fed anymore, but rather learning to feed themselves—and this requires foods that don't fall off or out of a spoon easily!

CUP-FEED

From around 6 months, babies can be taught to drink from an open cup. Use a teeny tiny cup like a little 30ml medicine cup or a shot glass. An adult needs to support the cup and control the flow of liquid. Start with a small volume such as 10ml (2 teaspoons) and tilt the cup so that the liquid, be it water or smoothie, moves to the edge and your baby can slurp it off. Be careful the contents aren't poured into your baby's mouth as they will likely cough and splutter. As they get better at controlling the movement of liquid from the cup to their mouth, you can put more in the cup and gradually reduce your external support. I had my daughter holding a 200ml cup and drinking independently (but closely supervised and not with a full cup) around 1 year old. She was great with a cup but terrible with straws—some kids will be the opposite. I will only use this type of drinking at her high chair, with water in cups/bottles with a non-spill valve everywhere else. Sippy cups and bottles that have the non-spill valves won't be appropriate to put smoothies in, because due to their increased viscosity, they are too hard to suck the smoothie out. If you remove the valve it may work okay, but it really depends on the size of the hole, so try it and see.

STRAWS

A lot of fun can be had with straws once your little one gets the hang of them. Despite persistence, my daughter didn't "get it" till after she was 1 year old, which was frustrating as I hoped it would be the main way I gave her smoothies. She was a very orally explorative child and she seemed to be teething her first teeth *forever*, so she would just bite on the straw whether it was a straw-sippy cup or an actual straw.

Options for straws are varied. Drink bottles with straws may come with a rigid, wider spout or a soft rubber straw, which will have a lid mechanism that bends it over and hides it, which is good for hygiene reasons while not in use. Some drinking cups come with lids that have a straw through them that may or may not move. Then you have plain straws that you put in an open cup. Straws may be single-use and disposable, such as plastic or paper ones, which also tend to be narrow. You can also get reusable straws made of stainless steel or glass, which are wider. The glass straws are made of tough glass like Pyrex, which is supposedly unbreakable—the one I bought has a lifetime guarantee on breakage.

Narrow straws will work facial muscles more, which is good for oral development, and wider ones can result in too much liquid being sucked up in one go. To avoid unnecessary waste, I don't recommend buying and disposing of plastic straws long term. The paper ones will at least biodegrade but they are still wasteful. I recommend teaching your baby to suck through a narrow straw, and once they have the hang of it and can control the suck and swallow required, switch to a reusable one, which tend to be wider.

With reusable straws, be very mindful of good hygiene. Like supply cups and straw cups, they need to be cleaned well in hot soapy water with a straw that is like a long, skinny bottle brush.

Around 9 months is the usual time that babies will be able to learn to use a straw, though many are capable much earlier. If they watch you use a straw often and are given the opportunity, they may well figure it out quickly. To get your baby used to the idea, dip a straw in 1 to 2 inches of water or milk, and place your thumb over the top to seal it. The liquid in the straw will stay there. Place the base of the straw in your baby's mouth and release your thumb from the other end so that the liquid goes in their mouth, if they happen to close their lips around the straw they will likely get the idea quicker. Do this a few times, then place the straw in a cup with just a little liquid and see if they suck it up. They will probably not master it the first time but repeat it a few times in a session. With persistence they should eventually get it. You may persist over just a few days if you are lucky, or it may be weeks, or in my case months! If they cough and sputter, use less liquid, a thinner straw, and/or try a thicker liquid that doesn't move as quickly as water, such as a smoothie or a smooth-fruit puree thinned with a little water or milk.

Smoothies drunk with a straw will be a separate straw in a cup. This will need external support by an adult for babies and probably for young toddlers too, particularly if there is not a lid on the cup that holds the straw in position.

ICE POPS

A brilliant way to feed smoothies to babies and kids is via homemade Popsicles, also known around the world as freeze pops, ice lollies, ice blocks, icy poles, chihiros, or ice pops. You can purchase specifically designed molds in all sorts of shapes and sizes or you can even use small cups that you stick an ice-cream stick into once partly frozen. Given kids and especially babies mouths are small, making ice pops that are skinny is sensible. This way it fits in your baby or toddler's mouth easily to suck on. As a bonus for babies and toddlers that are teething, a cold ice pop will be soothing to sore gums. Some ice pop molds have a handle that catch drips as it melts, with a spout off the handle to drink the drips up—very clever! You can turn any smoothie into an ice pop and you can do it with the intention to make a frozen meal or snack, or it's also a great way to freeze excess smoothie rather than it go to waste.

REUSABLE POUCHES

In recent years, purees and yogurts that come in pouches have become very popular as a meal on the go, as babies or toddlers can self-feed by sucking out the contents without the hassle and mess of feeding from open containers. However, for the small amount of food they contain they generate a lot of waste. Proponents of food pouches say they are better than buying jars because less heat is needed to cook the contents (less heat equals more nutrition), and because packaging is lighter it's more economical for transport. However, unlike the jars and lids of traditional processed baby food, which are handled by standard recycling programs, food pouches, apart from the caps, are not. Independent programs are in place in the United States, United Kingdom, and Australia to recycle the pouches, but without the convenience of adding them to your curbside collection, most end up in the trash and hence landfill. They are also an expensive way to feed your kids. For instance, looking at one brand in my supermarket that does the same yogurt in pouches, small tubs, and large tubs, I found that a small tub of the same weight as a pouch (120g) will cost half the price, and if buying a large tub (900g), per portion it's 2.6 times more expensive to buy the pouches. If making homemade yogurt it would be 6 to 16 times more expensive to use single-use pouches, depending on the milk you bought!

There is a solution that is best of both worlds—the convenience of a pouch without the environmental impact, and as an added bonus, it's your own food that goes into them, which is cheaper, and in most cases healthier. Many companies now sell such reusable pouches: In Australia, Sinchies and Little Mashies are well-known and reputable brands, Yummi Pouch and BooginHead Squeeze'Ems in the U.S. and My Pouch and Nom Nom Kids in the UK. Pouches will come in different sizes and are brilliant for smoothies—they can be filled fresh to drink that day or they can be frozen to thaw out and drink another day. Like reusable straws, it is very important that the pouches are cleaned and dried well to avoid contamination.

Dealing with Food Sensitivities

As discussed earlier, the current advice and scientific evidence states that no food needs to be withheld for reasons of avoiding food sensitivities. However, with 40 percent of children experiencing allergic sensitivities in countries such as the United States and Australia, awareness of reactions to foods is important. About 90 percent of reactions in infants are to egg or peanut, and whereas egg sensitivity tends to subside with time, peanut allergy is usually lifelong. In addition, 90 percent of food allergies are generally caused by the following foods: dairy, eggs, peanuts, soy, wheat, fish, crustacean shellfish, and tree nuts.

There are three ways our bodies are sensitive to foods: autoimmunity, allergies, and intolerances. These sensitivities have similar symptoms, though some are unique, as described below.

Autoimmune disorders involve an abnormal response by the immune system against normal substances and tissues in the body—essentially the body attacks itself. There are numerous autoimmune conditions that exist, including Hashimotos thyroiditis, type 1 diabetes, rheumatoid arthritis, and celiac disease. Furthermore, many autoimmune disorders coexist with celiac disease. Celiac disease is not an allergy, but a severe form of gluten intolerance that results in the lining of the intestines being anatomically altered, resulting in reduced ability to absorb nutrients from food into the bloodstream. Infants with celiac disease struggle to gain weight and height as expected and tend to be labeled "failure to thrive." Celiac disease may otherwise have no symptoms, but commonly associated symptoms are diarrhea, bloating, and skin rashes.

Allergies involve the immune system and are a result of the production of specific immunoglobulin, called IgE, to specific allergens. IgE-mediated allergies include hay fever, asthma, food allergy, insect venom allergy, latex allergy, and some drug allergies. The most common symptoms of food allergies include vomiting, diarrhea, blood in stools, eczema, hives, skin rashes, wheezing, and a runny nose. Other symptoms may include itchy lips/tongue/throat, stuffy nose, headaches, bellyache, diarrhea, gas, bloating, skin reactions, and sudden fatigue. Anaphylaxis is the most sudden and extreme reaction and is life threatening, with swelling of the throat and a drop in blood pressure that requires an injection of epinephrine. Symptoms are often immediate but may also be delayed. Skin prick testing is the primary method recommended for the diagnosis of IgE mediated allergies, with blood tests (RAST tests) sometimes done also.

Food intolerances are said to involve a delayed IgG or IgA response by the immune system and can occur hours to days later. Symptoms may include sore throat, mucous congestion, headaches, bellyaches, constipation, diarrhea, gas, bloating, hormone issues, foggy head, weight gain, fatigue, joint pain, depression, behavior changes, anxiety, and skin problems.

People with food sensitivities often know they are reacting to something they are eating and parents of children can tell you this much too, but it can be very difficult to tell what type of reaction is happening and to what—unless there is an obvious and immediate allergic reaction to something, such as eat an egg and vomit, or eat peanuts and stop breathing. It can also be difficult to pinpoint a problem food or foods, when many foods are eaten daily, or many times a day, such as wheat- or dairy-based foods, which if they are a problem then symptoms are just about constant.

If you suspect your child has a food sensitivity, then it is wise to get a referral from your family doctor to see a pediatric allergy specialist for testing. They will take a thorough history, choose which skin prick tests and/or blood tests to complete, and will advise you on the outcome.

In my daughter's case, I suspected that eggs in my diet were affecting her via my breast milk. She had multiple skin issues including a bad case of cradle cap, facial rashes, and eczema. She also fussed terribly at feed times, had green slimey poo, and vomited a lot. I had to breastfeed her small amounts often, and couldn't lay her flat for 20 to 30 minutes after a feed whether it was to play or sleep—it was exhausting! At 5 months I took eggs out of my diet and within 2 weeks her skin and fussing were 70 percent better. Meanwhile I had a referral sorted out for a specialist whom we saw at 8 months. My instinct told me not to introduce any nuts till we had her tested, which was lucky because both almonds and cashews came up positive, as well as wheat, egg yolk, and egg white. I was advised that it was not necessary for me to avoid these foods in my diet unless I was sure they reacted in hers—eggs we knew for sure but removing the nuts did help too.

They say they don't know yet why sensitivities develop in one person and not another. Clearly, my daughter was sensitized via my milk—eggs, almonds, and cashews are protein foods I ate a lot of while pregnant and breastfeeding. Wheat I don't eat, being gluten intolerant, but I did eat a little wheat accidentally when she was about 7 months old. I felt awful for 2 to 3 days and she was out of sorts too—so she was sensitized from that one exposure via my milk. I wonder whether my daughter's sensitivity stems from having to be on antibiotics for the first 2 weeks of her life and hence the impact on her gut flora? Or is it simply bad luck for her having two parents with sensitivities too? The genetic link is one thing they know makes developing sensitivities more likely. Very recent research, however, does point toward the impact of antibiotic use and the development of allergies, which suggests the importance of using probiotic therapy.

So in our case, there are no eggs or nuts in our diet including in our smoothies, and until around 1 year old my girl had an aversion to bananas, so smoothies for her were a challenge! Pears and blueberries were our saviors—she loves them both and as a bonus they are great sources of soluble fiber, so pooping is not a problem in my household!

While I advocate being professionally advised on what foods should and shouldn't be eaten in the case of sensitivities, if you suspect problems in your child, but it's not obvious about which food, and you are waiting to see a specialist, the smoothie-friendly foods that are least often associated with food allergies include apples, pears, sweet potatoes, cherries, carrots, and rice. All can be added to a smoothie cooked; sweet cherries and soft pears are the nicest and most appropriate to be added whole and raw. Carrots can be juiced and used as a liquid base, as well as rice milk, but do check the ingredients of commercial rice milk for quality and pick a calcium-enriched variety.

Dealing with Fussy Eaters

After all your hard work making healthy, tasty meals—be it a plate of food or a smoothie—the last thing you want to face is a child who won't eat it! There are many reasons why a child may be a fussy eater. It is suggested that there may be genetic predispositions to fussiness, such as some have sensory processing disorders that affect their tolerance of textured and new foods; or there may be developmental delay, associations with conditions such as autism, gut dysbiosis, behavioral problems such as hyperactivity, or they have been fed in a way that increases the risk of becoming fussy. Some things are relatively simple to remedy and others very complex and difficult.

DEFINING "FUSSY"

First, it's important to decide whether a child is actually "fussy." If a child has been highly stimulated by an activity or just been upset, and then plonked in a high chair and expected to eat a full meal and doesn't—are they truly fussy? Or are the circumstances surrounding their refusal to eat not their fault? Is a child who has been snacking all day, had a big lunch, or had a big glass of milk 30 minutes before dinner and then not interested in dinner really fussy? No, they are actually being sensible because they know they have eaten enough today—young children have an excellent ability to gauge the amount of calories they need in a day, much better than older children and adults. Is a child who won't "finish their plate" really fussy? Or is too much being put on their plate and they have simply eaten enough to satisfy their hunger? Is a child who refuses certain foods being fussy? It can take 10 to 15 presentations of the same food to a child before they eat it, and this is quite normal. Furthermore, infants may consistently refuse a food because they have a sensitivity to it.

Frequently, the label of "fussy" stems from a mismatch between the expectation of how much food a parent thinks a child should be eating and how much they actually need, particularly when a toddler's appetite slows as their growth rate slows in their second year, compared to being a hungry baby. Simply ensuring toddlers are not drinking more than 300ml to 500ml of milk over the day, and allowing toddlers to decide how much they want to eat, can make a huge difference at mealtimes. After 1 year old, toddlers without developmental problems should be mostly self-feeding anyway—by hand, with preloaded spoons/forks and learning to use a spoon and fork themselves. Don't offer a heap of food in one go; instead, offer a bit at a time and ideally a variety of things, and you will know when they have had enough as the food usually starts getting thrown on the floor, walls, or ceiling! If you put all the food available in front of them at once, it can overwhelm them and it may end up on the floor right away.

ALL CHILDREN ARE NOT THE SAME

Each child is different when it comes to eating, just like adults are different. Some people (and children) eat three main meals and little to no snacks, smaller meals and regular snacks, or larger meals *and* regular snacks. Understanding and respecting which works best will make for a happier family! In my mothers' group we have one girl who is a small eater, whereas my daughter is moderate and other children are huge eaters—and they are all thriving, happy, active, and healthy. My daughter will eat mostly at mealtimes and isn't much of a snacker (though at the time of writing this, I was still breastfeeding, so this may well change when I'm not breastfeeding anymore), and she will eat up to a cup of food, but not a cup of one food, more like a quarter cup each of four different foods.

If your child is a fan of smoothies, then they may well drink a cup or more in one go and that is their meal, or you may choose to have a small smoothie be part of a meal. It can be convenient to try and feed your child just one thing and hope they eat it all, but the reality is they probably won't, with both child and parent getting upset. Anyone who has fed a toddler knows that what they will eat one day, they may not the next for no apparent reason, and the volumes they eat can vary a lot too, so having a few food options available per meal is a good idea, and when you see the signs that they are done, respect that. As adults, we like a variety of food on our plate, too, and don't always finish what has been served up. When toddlers become very active, running around and learning about the world at a million miles per hour, getting them to stop for meals can be tricky. If this is the case with your toddler, allowing them to graze over the day eating mini-meals may suit them better. This is also a way to ensure they get enough calories and nutrition from their food without a battle ensuing at main mealtime because they don't want to sit still for long.

There are other simple strategies that can be used to avoid an unnecessary fussy label. Mealtimes should be calm—the child shouldn't be tired, upset, or stimulated by the TV. Snacks or big drinks, especially milk, should be avoided an hour before a meal. Never force-feed your baby such as sneaking spoons of food in. If your baby turns their head away or doesn't open their mouth to food, they don't want it or don't need it. Overfeed your baby and it will most likely end up on your carpet in the form of vomit. For older babies and younger toddlers, it can help to make sure food is ready and on the high-chair table as you put your child in, as this will be more successful in avoiding a protest.

Nutrition and Behavior

Children's food intake and behavior very much go hand in hand. Feed a child a high-glycemic diet, full of synthetic chemical additives, sugar, and bad fats, and not only will the child not be well nourished, but they will likely be more unsettled with play and sleep. Behavioral factors in turn can also negatively impact feeding. Many parents report that their toddlers are fussy eaters, with mealtimes a great source of stress. About 19 percent of mothers I surveyed were stressed/anxious about one or more of their children's fussy eating habits, and 74 percent of mothers had at least one fussy child. Out of the 21 options offered in my survey as strategies to improve eating habits of toddlers, all were well represented, suggesting parents are using a myriad of ideas to combat fussy eating, from less than ideal options such as nagging and bribery, to practical solutions such as being a good role model and eating with their child.

Human babies are born more immature than other mammals, with 90 percent of the growth of the human brain being in the first 5 years. The most immature part of the brain is the higher brain, which deals with reasoning and rationality. Also immature are the neural pathways joining the higher brain with the lower brain, which deals with emotions and socialization. The core or reptilian brain is all about basic instincts and survival. It's the reptilian brain that is doing most of the work with young babies. They don't understand the shades of gray in the world; it's all black or white: I am happy or I am not.

Nutrition and Hormones

Distress, anxiety, and fear trigger the release of cortisol from the adrenal glands. We know cortisol is a stress hormone. When gentle touch, care, and love are provided, oxytocin and opioids are released. We know that oxytocin is essential for the milk-ejection reflex in breastfeeding mothers. Oxytocin is a hormone of love—it is relaxing and makes you feel safe. Opioids are pain relieving and uplifting. Dopamine and serotonin are also hormones related to well-being. When these four substances are around we feel good; we feel comforted and loved; we are curious, motivated, and creative; and we have focus and are happy. Children and especially infants are extra vulnerable to the effects of junk food because of their immature brains and detoxification systems. Foods that contain sugar and additives such as artificial flavorings, colorings, and preservatives have a negative effect on the production of serotonin and dopamine, leading to bad behaviors such as hyperactivity, aggression, and being uncooperative, plus potential issues with poor sleep habits. On the flip side, certain foods can be used to boost serotonin and dopamine. The precursor to serotonin is the amino acid tryptophan and the precursor to dopamine is tyrosine. Serotonin helps keep you happy and calm while dopamine helps keep you alert and gives you drive. It's important to have both functioning, and a balanced plate of healthy food or smoothie can help supply the precursor amino acids vital to the production of these "feel good" hormones.

Smoothie-friendly sources of tryptophan: dairy, eggs, tahini, sunflower seeds, pumpkin seeds, almonds, fennel, celery, apricot, lettuce, carrot, bananas, spinach, kale, collards, oats, dates, and peanuts

Smoothie-friendly sources of tyrosine: spinach, dairy, almonds, peanuts, eggs, pumpkin seeds, avocados, and bananas

As you can see, these two amino acids exist in similar foods. Serve these regularly in smoothies alongside omega-3s in the diet, to optimize mood and mental health in your kids from a young age.

Dealing with Tantrums

Toddler tantrums can involve conflicts over food, and how to best deal with tantrums depends on the type of tantrum. Tantrums are best described as "distress tantrums" or "little Nero tantrums." With a distress tantrum the child is upset, crying, and incoherent. The immature brain cannot make sense of a situation such as separation from a loved one, or why they can't have something. They are not being naughty, should not be ignored, told off, or given time out, and trying to reason with them won't work. The child needs comfort and distraction. Uncomforted distress leads to higher levels of cortisol, which remains high even after they have calmed down. Little Nero tantrums, on the other hand, are characterized by a child being articulate without tears. The behavior is deliberate and a higher-brain action, and more typical of an older toddler or child. They are about power and control, and such tantrums if not dealt with properly while young may continue into childhood and adulthood and turn into "bullying" behavior. This behavior needs to be responded to with the message of "no," with time out used as a last resort. Negotiating, trying to reason, or offering comfort doesn't work.

A distress tantrum at mealtime may stem from a loved one leaving the house or from being taken away from playing. The distress needs to be settled with comfort before beginning or continuing the meal. In contrast, a child getting upset with a little Nero tantrum will make demands and not be happy not getting their way. Giving in may seem to keep the peace but in the long run, it doesn't help the child's character if they are the boss over the parents. This may also include demanding certain cups, specific foods, or continuing to play when it's mealtime. In these circumstances, parents need to be assertive about being in charge. Naturally, tantrums are best avoided in the first place, with the best approach to avoid triggers such as boredom, tiredness, frustration, tension, disappointment, and hunger. If any of these occur in the lead up to mealtime, then a frustrating mealtime for everyone can ensue.

If a child is on the verge of getting distressed, then distraction is the best method, such as singing to them while putting a bib on, and having food ready to go as soon as they sit down. If they are in the middle of an interesting play activity, assist to gently wind it up before calling them up for their meal. We don't like to be forced to stop what we are doing to "come and eat" as adults, and it's not fair to kids either.

Sugar and Mood

Problems with eating and behavior can come from the food being eaten itself. Foods and drinks that are high in sugar unopposed by fiber (e.g., fruit juice versus a fruit smoothie), processed foods high in sugar, and processed carbohydrates such as white bread and cookies will result in a spike in blood sugar followed by a sudden drop. This can manifest as hyperactivity in a child followed by moody behavior—no different from the effects of swings in blood sugar in adults. A child who consistently wants carbs and sweet foods and drinks (as opposed to going through phases, which is pretty normal for many toddlers) may have an underlying issue with their gut health, namely dysbiosis—an imbalance of good and bad bacteria in the form of candida overgrowth. The prolific sugars supplied by the diet feed the candida and they proliferate further, demanding more sugar to feed off, and hence a vicious cycle emerges. According to Dr. Natasha Campbell-McBride, the author of *Gut and Psychology Syndrome* (or GAPS), this scenario is common in children (and adults) with significant behavioral problems, such as autism, ADHD, ADD, dyslexia, dyspraxia, and even schizophrenia and depression. Dr. Campbell-McBride reversed her child's autism by following the program she developed that essentially removes processed foods, grains (especially gluten), dairy, and sugars from the diet, and uses whole foods, bone broths, and probiotics to heal the gut. Even without the obvious existence of one of these disorders, if your child consistently wants only carbs and sweet foods and drinks, they may have a candida overgrowth issue and would benefit from a protocol to get it under control. Such dietary fussiness is highly likely to go hand in hand with problem behavior, so working with an appropriate health professional to guide the process is recommended.

IRON DEFICIENCY

Other food-related reasons for fussiness can include iron deficiency, which is a bit of a double-edged sword because you need food to supply iron, but iron deficiency can reduce appetite. About 6.6 percent to 15.2 percent (depending on ethnicity) of toddlers in the United States are reported to be iron deficient. If your infant is iron deficient, or you suspect they are, then ensure what they do eat is iron-rich and seek professional advice in case supplementation is required as well. Also, remember that vitamin C helps with iron absorption and vitamin A helps release stored iron, so a smoothie that contains iron, vitamin A, and vitamin C together is sensible. Vitamins A and C are generally abundant in fresh fruit, particularly green, yellow, orange, and red fruits. As previously discussed, iron and calcium compete for absorption, so very rich sources of calcium such as cow's milk are best avoided or minimized in the same meal as iron-rich foods, particularly for infants with iron deficiency and for babies from 6 to 12 months, whose iron requirement is higher than that of a toddler. This is the reason why cow's milk is not recommended as a drink for babies, but can be used sparingly in cooking and in cereal. I would consider cow's milk in a smoothie "a drink" by this definition and recommend it be minimized, alongside servings of yogurt over a couple of tablespoons.

Smoothie-friendly iron sources for children: leafy greens (especially spinach, chard, and parsley), dried apricots, figs, raspberries, raisins, prunes, beets, tahini, turmeric, pumpkin seeds, hemp seeds, quinoa, and eggs

The Importance of Nutrient-Dense Foods

Touched on earlier is the point that a toddler's growth rate slows in comparison to a baby's. You can see this on growth charts that are almost vertical in the first few months and gradually flatten out with time. In the absence of a medical problem causing fussy eating, one theory why toddlers frequently have an aversion to vegetables is that they fill them up without satisfying them. Vegetables, though nutritious, are for the most part high in water and fiber and low in calories—a perfect food for adults to fill up on with their much larger stomachs, but for little tummies it's best to go for nutrient-dense foods such as concentrated proteins and fats. In smoothies these foods include nuts, seeds, avocado, yogurt, and greens.

Greens in particular are a great way of getting the nutrients into toddlers that veggies do, but with much less volume. If your toddler develops an aversion to veggies and greens visually before even eating them, then hiding them is the usual approach parents take, though many kids can tell and can see the teeny tiniest fleck of zucchini in a sauce! This is where smoothies are just fabulous at hiding things, as it's all blended nice and smoothly. Then being creative with how the smoothie looks and tastes is the next challenge. In my survey, 70 percent of mothers who had given smoothies to their young children needed to use strategies to encourage their consumption. Successful solutions included the use of colored or non-transparent cups, adding milk or yogurt to make smoothies creamier, disguising color with the use of berries or cacao, ensuring combinations are sufficiently sweet, and creating smoothies that are super smooth. The suggestion that adding greens to smoothies is too hard on the digestion for little ones was not supported by my survey with only 4 percent reporting this to be the case.

Based on my research and my experience, the following is a summary of what I think works to combat fussy eating or potentially fussy eating:

Associate food and eating with fun. This is especially useful with babies and younger toddlers. Use colored and patterned plates, bowls, cups, and utensils. Encourage playing with food and allow mess to happen without tidying up along the way.

Don't punish poor eating nor reward good eating. Then your child isn't made to feel like they have been naughty and you don't get caught up in the giving of treats.

Avoid being in your child's face. Having someone stare at you while you eat would put us off as adults, wouldn't it? Keep your distance and keep an eye on them for safety but let them get on with it.

Be a good role model. Explain what foods are as you prepare them and serve them. Try and eat with your child and let them see you eat a variety of foods.

Lower your expectations. You need to lower your expectations of how much you think they need to be eating. Offer food bit by bit and respect when they don't want to eat anymore. Understand that amounts will vary meal to meal and day to day. And never force-feed your child.

Progress into textures. If starting with pureed food, progress fairly quickly into lumpier and textured food, especially by 7 months. Introduce finger foods by at least 9 months and aim to have your baby eating family food, not baby food, around 1 year old. Smoothies are an exception as they will always need to be very smooth, which is how they should be anyway—they are called smoothies after all!

Offer as much variety as you can. This should be done before your baby turns 1, before their growth rate and appetite reduce in their second year.

Aim to provide food that is nutritious in every mouthful. "Empty-calorie" snacks such as rice crackers and sweets, and overconsumption of bread products, is counterproductive to healthy eating habits.

Avoid situations where your child is upset before or at mealtime. Work on calming them down before you try and feed them—unless they are super hungry, then give them something as soon as possible, like a piece of finger food.

Keep mealtimes calm. If your child is aroused or anxious this will decrease their appetite, so make mealtimes relatively calm. This includes your behavior. If you are agitated or anxious, your child will pick up on this.

Smoothies for Babies and Toddlers

In terms of volumes of smoothie to feed your kids, it's best to be guided by them. According to my survey, these were the most common volumes drunk by age:

- Babies: less than ½ cup
- Toddlers 1 to 3 years: ½ cup
- Toddlers 4 to 5 years: 1 cup
- Mothers: 1½ to 2 cups

Smoothies being made for both parents only made up 15 percent of respondents in my survey, and partners were more likely to have a smoothie as a snack, versus mothers mostly having them as a meal. My survey also revealed that a number of older toddlers drank less than half a cup, and some younger toddlers drank more than 2 cups. The following recipes will make 2 cups. This will be an average amount for a parent and infant to share, an amount that may well suit feeding more than one child, or enough for multiple infant servings, with leftovers saved for the next day or frozen into reusable food pouches, or made into Popsicles or ice cubes. If you need more smoothie than 2 cups, then adapt the recipe.

In a nutshell, a smoothie for older babies and toddlers should be nutrient dense, focusing on protein, good fats, iron, zinc, vitamins A and C, and calcium. Ideally, use a liquid with nutrients like milk or coconut water, and avoid too much fiber such as using celery, chia seeds, and lots of raw greens or non-sweet vegetables. These foods are low calorie and filling for little tummies, discouraging weight gain.

It is also advised to try to make them creamy, naturally sweet, super smooth, and not too watery, and in some cases it is advised to disguise the color. Recipes will focus on these main points. If you are currently breastfeeding, your nutrient requirements are very high, so it's important that smoothies you consume are well designed for your needs (as explained in Chapter 5, "After the Baby Is Born"), particularly if you need smoothies that promote lactation. The priority nutrients for infants and lactating women are somewhat similar, and thus there are recipes that will suit both groups simultaneously. However, ingredients such as honey, herbal teas, raw eggs, protein powders, cacao, and chia, which are suitable for lactation, are not suitable for babies. Honey can be used after a child is 1 year old, and raw eggs and cacao may be used cautiously with toddlers, as previously discussed in this chapter. Protein powders are too concentrated for young children and may provide too much protein in their diets, so better to get protein from whole foods.

Please note that recipes will vary in thickness and sweetness according to the choice of ingredients, and this will vary further, particularly with flavor, due to differences between seasons and produce quality. Should a recipe turn out thicker than you would like, add some more liquid; if it's not sweet enough, add some sweetener; if you like cold smoothies, use some ice in place of the liquid component. If you haven't read the introductory chapters before attempting my recipes, please go back and read them, particularly Chapter 1, "The Art and Science of Smoothies," which has detailed guidelines for my smoothie creations.

All recipes in this chapter yield 2 cups (500ml) that serve mother and baby or multiple infants.

BABIES' FIRST SMOOTHIES

If you plan to start your baby on smoothies when they first start solids, start very simply with 1 to 2 ingredients only plus liquid. Bear in mind your young baby will likely only eat a few teaspoons to start with, and even if they work their way up to a few tablespoons over their first months or so, that still isn't much smoothie and you aren't going to blend up a teeny tiny portion! My suggestion is to make the base of a smoothie for you—remove a portion for them and then add more ingredients into your smoothie. Take out more than they will eat to account for spillage, about a quarter cup.

Choose one or two ingredients from the list of fruits and vegetables below totaling 1½ cups (please note any cooked ingredients are cooled before use):

- Banana (ripe enough that skin is all yellow plus getting brown spots)

- Papaya (red is nicer)

- Pear (soft and ripe, or steamed or stewed)

- Mango (ensure it is ripe so it is sweet)

- Blueberries (frozen work well and are less expensive)

- Melon (pair with blueberries only or on its own)

- Peaches (soft and ripe, or steamed or stewed)

- Apricots (soft and ripe, or steamed or stewed)

- Apple (steamed or stewed)

- Carrot (steamed)

- Sweet potato (steamed)

- Pumpkin (steamed)

- Coconut (fresh and soft flesh from a drinking coconut)

- Avocado (¼ cup maximum and pair with any of the above except melon)

1. Add ¾ cup of filtered water, coconut water, coconut milk, almond milk, rice milk, formula, or breast milk.

2. Blend till smooth.

3. Remove ¼ cup or less for baby.

4. Store the rest as described above or use as a base for your own smoothie.

Example

> ¾ cup mango
>
> ¾ cup papaya
>
> ¾ cup coconut water
>
> This can be used as a base for the Papaya and Mango Mender recipe on page 209.
>
> ¾ cup mango
>
> ¾ cup papaya
>
> ¾ cup coconut water
>
> 2 tablespoons hemp seeds
>
> 1 teaspoon vanilla extract or paste, or ½ vanilla bean
>
> handful of spinach (optional)

The following smoothies from the recipe section in Chapter 5, "After the Baby Is Born," are also suitable for this purpose, i.e., the have a base of simple baby-friendly ingredients. I have added a 🥕 next to each of these recipes in that chapter.

- Sweet Satisfaction (page 206)

- Gimme a Boost (page 207)

- Coco-Banana Passion (page 208)

- Apricot Tart (page 209)

- Banana and Protein Punch (page 210)

- Peaceful Papaya (page 211)

- Spicy Sweet Potato (page 211)

- Merry Milky Mango (page 213)

- Berry and Banana Blessings (page 215)

- Spiced Pumpkin and Banana Brew (page 217)

- Melon and Passion Fruit Pleasure (just blend melon and no extra liquid) (page 218)

- Summer Love (page 218)

- Papaya and Lime Lift (page 217)

- Spicy Pear and Pumpkin (page 227)

- Motherly Mango (page 227)

- Fearless Fennel and Chocolate (page 228)

Once your baby has tried a wider variety of foods both in smoothies and in their diet generally, including grains, fruits, veggies, nuts, seeds, and different types of milk, they can have more adventurous smoothies.

SMOOTHIE RECIPES FOR OLDER BABIES (8 TO 12 MONTHS)

While dairy milk may be consumed by older babies, it should not be their main source of milk—this should be breast milk or formula. Because iron and calcium compete with each other in the body for absorption, it is recommend to minimize dairy consumption (milk and yogurt) before a child is 1 year old. Many of the recipes list "any milk" in the ingredient list. This may include cow's milk but please don't use cow's milk for every smoothie you make, particularly if making them daily. Offer a variety of milks or use coconut water instead.

The following smoothie recipes designed for older babies are also suitable for toddlers.

Banana Pudding

1 banana, fresh or frozen and sliced

¾ cup red papaya or mango

¾ cup any milk or coconut water

1 tablespoon hemp or sunflower seeds*

small handful of spinach (optional)

*Ideally, soak sunflower seeds overnight in water, then drain and rinse before use—this will aid digestibility and help them blend smoothly. However, avoid sunflower seeds if you don't have a high-speed blender, as kids won't like a smoothie that isn't smooth, with small bits of seeds through it.

Peachy Berry Bliss

1 cup halved peaches (soft and ripe or steamed)

½ cup raspberries or strawberries

½ cup any milk or coconut water

2 tablespoons full-fat natural yogurt

1 teaspoon vanilla paste

Blue Bananas

1 banana

¾ cup frozen blueberries

¾ cup any milk or coconut water

¼ avocado

handful of spinach (optional)

Pineapple Pop

¾ cup cantaloupe

¾ cup pineapple

1 medium Persian cucumber

few mint leaves (optional)

Nutty Nanas

1 banana

¾ cup nectarine or plum halves*

¼ cup coconut flesh from a drinking coconut

¾ cup any milk or coconut water

pinch of ground Sri Lankan cinnamon

*It's essential that fresh stone fruit are ripe, sweet, and juicy.

Melon Mania

1 cup honeydew melon

1 large or 2 small soft, raw pears, quartered

handful of leafy greens such as kale, spinach, or Swiss chard (optional)

Apple Pie

½ cup cooked oats, quinoa, or millet

¾ cup steamed pear or apple

½–1 tablespoon nut butter

¼ teaspoon ground Sri Lankan cinnamon

1 cup almond milk

Kiwi Kracker

2 cups watermelon (ensure it's a seedless variety or remove the seeds)

1 kiwi, without skin

Creamy Porridge

½ cup cooked oats, quinoa, or millet

1 banana

¼ avocado

1 cup any milk

1 medjool date, pitted, or 2 prunes, pitted

1 teaspoon vanilla paste

Mango Berry Blast-Off

¾ cup mango

¾ cup raspberries or strawberries

¼ cup natural yogurt plus ½ cup milk, or ¾ cup milk kefir

Pumpkin Pie

½ cup sweet potato, carrot, or pumpkin puree

1 banana, fresh or frozen and sliced

1 cup any milk

pinch of ground Sri Lankan cinnamon

few leaves baby bok choy (optional)

Kermit the Frog

1 cup fresh figs, stem tip removed

¾ cup seedless grapes

¾ cup almond milk

6 raw walnut or pecan halves*

handful of spinach (optional)

*Ideally, soak overnight, drain, and rinse before blending.

Purple Princess/Prince

½ cup cooked oats, quinoa, or millet

¾ cup berries, cherries, or mixture

2 heaping tablespoons diced raw or steamed beet

½ cup coconut water

2 tablespoons full-fat natural yogurt or ¼ cup flesh from a drinking
coconut

Marvelous Mandarins

1 packed cup mandarin segments

1 cup raw, steamed, or pureed pears*

1–2 tablespoons hemp seeds

*The gritty texture of raw pears in a smoothie is reduced by the cooking process,
and may be better tolerated by your older baby.

Is It Orange or Blue?

1 cup freshly squeezed orange juice

1½ cups frozen blueberries

½–1 tablespoon hulled tahini

handful of lettuce or spinach

SMOOTHIES FOR TODDLERS (AGES 1 TO 3)

Once your baby turns 1 and is officially a toddler, you can start using honey as a sweetener in small amounts and in moderation as it is a form of concentrated sugar.

The use of dairy can be more relaxed as the iron requirements of toddlers (7mg per day) is less than that of an older baby (11mg per day); hence, calcium-rich dairy milk and yogurt won't be as much of an issue with its competition for iron absorption. Additionally, calcium requirements for a toddler almost double to 500mg per day. Therefore, where "any milk" is listed in recipes below, dairy may be used as often as you wish. Dairy of course doesn't need to be the primary source of calcium, especially if still breastfeeding. But if not, calcium can be supplied from many other suitable smoothie-friendly sources including green leafy vegetables, tahini, almonds, figs, and oats—not to mention calcium from non-smoothie meals in the diet.

The careful and hygienic use of raw eggs may also be used in smoothies for children at 1 year old. Only reputable sources of eggs should be used (organic/chemical-free and grass-eating free range), they should be fresh, the shell washed, and each egg checked before putting in your smoothie—it should not smell, the white should not be watery, and the yolk should not break easily. The risk of salmonella from "conventionally farmed" raw eggs is 1 in 30,000, so risk is low, and even lower and likely negligible with ethical eggs.

The following recipes make approximately 2 cups, which may be the volume a hungry toddler drinks, or more likely a volume split between siblings, shared between parent and child, portioned and stored for the next day, or frozen into pouches or ice-pop molds. With a fussy toddler, consider the need to disguise smoothie colors (e.g., green) in an opaque cup with a lid or add berries to change the color, or focus on colorful smoothies, e.g., gorgeous bright pink or yellow ones. Moreover, it's enjoyable to make up funny names for smoothies and when children are talking, get them involved with making up names, too.

Monkey Magic

1 banana, frozen and sliced or fresh

¾ cup red papaya or mango

¾ cup any milk or coconut water

1 tablespoon hemp or sunflower seeds*

small handful of spinach (optional)

1 egg (optional)

*Ideally, soak sunflower seeds overnight in water, then drain and rinse before use—this will aid digestibility and help them blend smoothly. However, avoid sunflower seeds if you don't have a high-speed blender, as kids won't like a smoothie that isn't smooth, with small bits of seeds through it.

Prince Caspian's Pineapple

¾ cup cantaloupe

¾ cup pineapple

1 medium Persian cucumber

few mint leaves (optional)

Princess Anna's Apricots

¾ cup steamed peaches or apricots

¾ cup raspberries or strawberries

½ cup any milk or coconut water

¼ cup coconut flesh from a drinking coconut or 2 tablespoons coconut cream

1 teaspoon vanilla paste

1 egg (optional)

Peter Pan's Pumpkins

½ cup steamed or pureed sweet potato or pumpkin

1 cup orange or mandarin orange segments

½–1 tablespoon peanut butter (or other nut/seed butter)

¾ cup almond milk

3 medjool dates, pitted, or 6 prunes, pitted

1 teaspoon vanilla paste

Ka-Pow!

½ cup cooked oats, quinoa, or millet

1 banana, fresh or frozen and sliced

1 cup any milk

1 heaping teaspoon raw cacao

½–1 tablespoon any nut butter

3 medjool dates, pitted

pinch of ground nutmeg

handful of kale or other brassica (optional)

The Batmobile

1 fresh banana

¾ cup frozen blueberries

¾ cup any milk or coconut water

¼ avocado or ¼ cup full-fat natural yogurt

handful of spinach (optional)

1 medjool date, pitted

1 egg (optional)

Bananas in Pajamas

1 banana, fresh or frozen and sliced

¾ cup nectarine or plum halves*

8 cashews or 6 macadamias

¾ cup any milk or coconut water

pinch of ground Sri Lankan cinnamon

1 egg (optional)

*It's essential that fresh stone fruit are ripe, sweet, and juicy.

Green Goblin

½ cup raw muesli soaked in 1½ cups milk overnight in the fridge

handful of leafy greens such as kale, spinach, or Swiss chard

Pink Panther

1 cup watermelon (ensure it's a seedless variety or remove the seeds)

1 kiwi, without skin, halved

¾ cup frozen strawberry halves

Big Bird's Breakfast

½ cup cooked oats, quinoa, or millet

1 banana, fresh or frozen and sliced

¼ avocado

1 medjool date, pitted, or 2 prunes, pitted

1 teaspoon vanilla paste

1 cup any milk

1 egg (optional)

Strawberries and Cream

½ cup cooked oats, quinoa, or millet

1½ cups/1 punnet strawberries with hulls

1 tablespoon raw beet*

3 medjool dates, pitted

1 teaspoon vanilla paste

*The beet will give this smoothie a nice pink color and won't affect the taste.

SpongeBob's Pear and Porridge Pie

½ cup cooked oats, quinoa, or millet

¾ cup steamed pear or apple

½–1 tablespoon nut butter

¼ teaspoon ground Sri Lankan cinnamon

1 cup almond milk

1 egg (optional)

A Cup of Sunshine

½ cup mango flesh

½ cup steamed or raw carrot

3 tablespoons coconut cream

1 teaspoon vanilla paste

1 cup any milk

thin slice fresh ginger (optional)

Bert and Ernie's Berries

¾ cup mango

¾ cup raspberries or strawberries

¼ cup natural yogurt plus ½ cup milk, or ¾ cup milk kefir

1 egg (optional)

The Gingerbread House

½ cup steamed or pureed sweet potato or pumpkin

1 banana, fresh or frozen and sliced

¼-inch slice fresh ginger

2 dried figs with stem tips removed, soaked in 1 cup of any milk overnight in the fridge

1 tablespoon hemp seeds

Spicy Superman/Superwoman

½ cup cooked oats, quinoa, or millet

¼ cup sweet potato, carrot, or pumpkin puree

¾ cup any milk

¼ teaspoon ground Sri Lankan cinnamon

1 teaspoon vanilla paste

little honey or maple syrup to taste

few leaves baby bok choy (optional)

1 egg (optional)

Purple People Eater

½ cup cooked oats, quinoa, or millet

¾ cup berries, pitted cherries, or mixture

2 tablespoons raw diced beet

¾ cup coconut water

1 egg (optional)

Ready, Steady, Wiggle

1 packed cup mandarin orange segments

1 cup fresh pineapple pieces

1 tablespoon hemp seeds

1 teaspoon vanilla paste

Ben 1 0's Blueberry Juice

1 cup freshly squeezed orange juice

1½ cups frozen blueberries

½–1 tablespoon hulled tahini

handful of lettuce or spinach (optional)

FEATURED SMOOTHIES

The following recipes are some wonderful contributions by mothers around the world—tried and tested recipes used by families who love smoothies and some who have had kids on the fussy side.

Alexx Stuart's Recipes

Alexx Stuart is the author of the Amazon bestseller *Real Treats*, an e-book full of guilt-free treats that are gluten- and refined-sugar-free. Alexx is an avid researcher and recipe creator for her website alexxstuart.com and her online course, 30 Days to Your Low-Tox Life.

Alexx says: Feeding my little guy was such a joy in those toddler years, as he discovered tastes, textures, and flavors. From 18 months old he had as much of a say as I did about which fruits and vegetables we had at home and I truly believe my taking him to markets at this age, along with my enthusiastic tone for fresh produce, has helped him continue to be a kid who just LOVES veggies and fruit. I always say, if we used as much enthusiasm for zucchini toward our kids as we did when we offered them a cupcake, fussy eating wouldn't exist. We always seem to, as a culture, sound "cross" with our kids, hurrying them up to eat all their vegetables—if we make it SOUND like a chore, then they'll think pretty quickly that it is one. One of the yummiest ways to get kids in the kitchen of course is blending up various smoothie creations—the following recipes were created at random over the years, as much by my son, as by me. A team effort!

Alexx's recipes yield 2 cups.

Berry Coconut Lime Cheesecake Smoothie

1 cup berries (frozen or fresh)

1 cup coconut milk (or half coconut cream/half water)

juice of 1 lime

1 tablespoon maple syrup or rice malt syrup

Super Speedy Choc-Banana "Thick Shake" Smoothie

This is THE perfect recipe for a fussy child or an active, growing, sporty toddler who needs the fuel.

2–3 teaspoons raw cacao powder

2 teaspoons honey, or maple or rice syrup

1 cup milk of your choice

¼ cup coconut cream

½ avocado

½ teaspoon ground cinnamon

Cool as a Cucumber Smoothie

1 Persian cucumber

2 kiwi or 1 apple, quartered

½ cup coconut water

handful of mint leaves

Franki's Recipes

Franki is a mother of three and her kids love green smoothies.

Frankie says: My kids are 8, 6, and 3 and all enjoy their "Shrek juice." Especially the 3-year-old, who is always finished first and asks for more. He is having this green smoothie regularly because he is going through that fussy stage where he likes to say no to lots of food, but he never says no to "Shrek juice." I like to keep sliced bananas and avocados and chopped kale in the freezer so I've always got these ingredients on hand.

Franki's recipes yield 3 cups that serve 2 to 3 kids or an adult and a child.

Shrek Juice

1 cup coconut water

1 banana

½ cup kale

½ avocado

1 date, pitted

Jo Whitton's Recipes

Jo Whitton, a mother of five and the author of *Quirky Cooking* and the website quirkycooking.com.au, Jo has been recognized as a top Australian food blogger and is a sought-after presenter of her quirky style of cooking, which is influenced by health problems experienced by her and her children that have led her to create delicious allergy-friendly recipes.

Jo says: My mum taught me to cook from a very young age, using basic, fresh ingredients, and cooking "from scratch." I developed an interest in healthy eating as I grew up, and when I got married and we started our own family, I worked hard to cook wholesome, delicious meals. Healthy eating doesn't have to be boring. Food intolerances and allergies don't have to make life difficult. My hope is that *Quirky Cooking* will help to open people's eyes to the possibility of wholesome food that tastes great, is easy and fun to make, and meets the needs of those with diet challenges.

I love the vibrant colors of smoothies made with fresh fruits and greens. When my kids were little, I taught them to love green smoothies by calling them things like "green monster smoothies." Make it fun, and kids will love it. And if all else fails and you just can't get them to drink something that's green, pour it into a kid's reusable squeezie pouch that they can't see through. You can hide just about anything in those cute little pouches, and kids love them!

Jo's recipes yield 4 cups (1 liter) that serve 2.

. . . .

Creamy Pine-Lime Green Smoothie

¾ cup raw cashews

1 apple, quartered

1 large orange, peeled and halved

1 lime, peeled

1 cup frozen pineapple cut in 1-inch cubes

handful of baby spinach leaves

1½ cups unsweetened coconut water

Susan's Recipe

Susan's son has just turned 1 and they both love smoothies.

Susan says: In addition to the convenience of making smoothies for myself in the mornings, I have also introduced my son to smoothies for breakfast. Unfortunately, he isn't the best eater, so if he doesn't eat much else during the day, he has at least had a really good breakfast with lots of vitamins, minerals, fats, and protein in his smoothie. I love that the couple of times that he has had a cold I was able to add things like pumpkin seeds for zinc and oranges and lemons for vitamin C to the smoothie, to help support his immune system. It was pretty messy to begin with trying to feed him the smoothie from a cup, but since he has learned to drink from a straw, it has made breakfast time much neater, easier, and quicker, given he no longer tries to tip the container upside down! So we can leave the house earlier following breakfast or he can have his smoothie after we leave.

I tend to make up my recipes as I go along, but this is an example of an effective immune-boosting smoothie that my son loved.

Susan's recipe yields 3 cups that serves a mother and a child.

½ peeled orange

¼ peeled lemon

1 tablespoon pumpkin seeds

1 tablespoon hemp seeds

¼ avocado

½ Persian cucumber

¼ inch slice zucchini

1 cup coconut water

½ teaspoon vanilla extract

maple syrup to taste

Kira's Recipe

Kira Westwick is the author of the book *Wholesome Kids*, was on *MasterChef Australia* in 2014, and she combines her love for family, food, and fitness at kirawestwick.com.au. Kira believes that life is to be lived energetically and joyfully, without deprivation, especially when it comes to food!

Kira says: Smoothies are an ideal tool for helping children fall in love with whole foods. Creating consistently healthy, convenient, and kid-friendly meals each day can be challenging. That is why I always have a supply of smoothie ingredients on hand, so I can whip up a dense and nutritious snack at a moment's notice that I know my kids will devour! Homemade smoothies really are the most convenient and delightful way to ensure children get the recommended daily servings of fresh fruits and vegetables essential for optimal growth, concentration, and development. Have fun naming smoothies with your children—they can suddenly become very appealing if they are going to make them "super strong like Ben 10" or "give them shiny hair like a princess!" Choose something desirable and relevant to your child. Also, serve smoothies up in style—children are more likely to give something a go if it looks fun and engaging! And always add a straw for a smooth drinking experience.

Kira's recipe yields 4 cups (1 liter).

Sunshine Smoothie

This smoothie can transform your "picky" eater into a healthy-food connoisseur!

1 medium cucumber, quartered

1 handful of sunflower sprouts or spinach

1 orange, peeled and halved

1 apple, cut into 8 pieces

1 cup filtered water

½ cup ice

Alison's Recipe

Alison is a mama of two and a lover of smoothies. While breastfeeding her youngest, she made smoothies with almond milk, chia, bananas, avocado, nutmeg, and vanilla, which helped boost her afternoon milk supply.

Alison says: Since my baby was around 7 to 8 months, I have been making her a smoothie for lunch. The family loves it so much they all come around when feeding her to see if there are leftovers that they can snatch. I also pop in her baby probiotic powder with it, and if there is inflammation such as teething or diaper rash, I also pop in half a cucumber for its cooling effects.

Alison's recipe yields 4 cups (1 liter) that serves the whole family.

1 banana

½ avocado

1 cup cantaloupe or peaches

1½ cups of water, or 1 cup water

½ Persian cucumber

Bianca Slade's Recipe

Bianca Slade of wholefoodsimply.com is a mother of two, aged 2 and 6, and has published three cookbooks with gorgeous photography and beautiful personal stories alongside her creations.

Bianca says: I am not entirely sure how Wholefood Simply came to be. Perhaps it all started many years ago when my journey into clean eating began. Perhaps it was much later than that, when I had a baby of my own and noticed how many children were eating processed and packaged foods. Today, my aim is to make things a little easier for those who are embarking on the real-foods path. I want to help families who live with intolerances and allergies. I want to put fun and simplicity into what can sometimes be a daunting and dull experience. Ultimately, I want to create food that is enjoyed by all.

My little boy is fussy, and smoothies made with fruits and vegetables have been an integral part of his diet. I cannot begin to tell you how good this smoothie is! Our "Jar of Pumpkin and Pecan Pie" is pure comfort food! Rich, thick, heavy, and warming, it is also sweet, hearty, and tastes almost sinful. My toddler drank all of his, and then pinched his sister's!

Bianca's recipe yields 3 cups.

A Jar of Pumpkin and Pecan Pie

1 frozen banana, sliced

1 cup cold roast pumpkin or pumpkin puree

handful of pecans

1 teaspoon ground cinnamon

1 cup water

Sarah's Recipe

Sarah is a chiropractor and mother of two, aged 4 and 5.

Sarah says: I'm a big believer that children learn through example. We have no packaged foods in our house and every mealtime is an opportunity to teach and demonstrate good nutritional decisions and eating. My 4-year-old is incredible in the decisions she makes with food when out and about, even at birthday parties. When they were just starting solids, though, and might not have loved a new food, we would throw it into a smoothie. My theory was to allow their body to start to recognize and receive the benefits of the food without them having to necessarily look at it. After a week or so of doing this, I often found they would then enjoy the food in its whole form.

My kids definitely love banana-based smoothies at breakfast. Sometimes if they turn their nose up at a green smoothie, I camouflage the identical one by adding cacao and some frozen berries and calling it a choc-berry smoothie! The following recipe is a favorite in our house and a taste sensation!

Sarah's recipe yields 2 cups and serves 2 toddlers.

Carrot Cake Smoothie

- 1 cup frozen banana, sliced
- ¼ inch slice fresh ginger
- ½ cup carrot juice
- ½ cup almond milk
- ½ teaspoon ground cinnamon
- ¼ vanilla bean

Amy's Recipe

Amy is a busy mother of three young boys who love their afternoon smoothies.

Amy says: Our after-school smoothie came about after my 9-year-old's favorite vegan ice cream. We loved the flavors so we decided to try them all in a smoothie as afternoon tummy filler. YUM! With three boys that are always hungry, my younger being nearly 2, I find this keeps them out of the pantry, especially in the afternoon when they are always "starving"!

Amy's recipe yields 3 cups and serves 3 children.

Better Than Ice Cream Smoothie

1 cup frozen banana, sliced

1 tablespoon nut butter

1-2 teaspoons raw cacao

1-2 teaspoons maple syrup

2 cups almond milk or oat milk

Kelly's Recipe

Kelly is a mama of two, aged 2 and 4, and has had very mixed results feeding her kids smoothies.

Kelly says: With my son, I think I started too late trying to give him smoothies and he won't have a bit of it, and he is very sensitive to flavors such as coconut. My daughter on the other hand has smoothies with me all the time and she frequently walks around with her mason jar of smoothie.

Kelly's recipe yields 4 cups (1 liter) that serves the whole family.

Dragon's Blood Smoothie

flesh from 1 mango

1 frozen banana, sliced

1 Persian cucumber, quartered

1 lime, peeled

1-2 handfuls kale or spinach

1 cup coconut water

Sarah's Recipe

Sarah is a mother of three children, aged 2, 4, and 9.

Sarah says: My husband and I overhauled our family's eating habits when one of our children developed a lot of digestive problems, and we have had fantastic results with a whole-food, low-grain lifestyle, which includes smoothies and juices each morning. The following recipe is a favorite of our kids. It makes around a liter of smoothie, so it feeds all of us!

Sarah's recipe yields 4 cups (1 liter) that serves the whole family.

. . . .

Piña Colada

flesh and water from a drinking coconut

2 cups fresh pineapple pieces

1 banana, frozen and sliced

Gabriela Rosa's Recipe

Gabriela Rosa is a proud mama of her 2½-year-old son, fertility specialist, and author and founder of www.NaturalFertility Breakthrough.com.

Gabriela says: He must be an anomaly! If it's food, Jake will eat it. He eats and drinks everything and loves his smoothies! I've always been a big fan of smoothies; in fact my mother raised my sister and I on them. I think that I have had smoothies for breakfast since I began eating and that is pretty much what I have done with Jake. The following recipe is one of my family's favorite. I blend it for about 1½ minutes to ensure it is really smooth, and the beet gives it a lovely bright pink color that Jake loves, and he regularly asks for a "pink smoothie"! Essentially you can use any vegetables you have in the house; it will all be deliciously disguised with the help of the other ingredients. I even successfully sneak them into my lovely husband's smoothie!

Gabriela's recipe yields 4 cups (1 liter) that serves the whole family.

. . . .

Jake's Pink Smoothie

½ cup raw oats

1 banana

100g frozen berries

handful of nuts (your choice—cashews are lovely)

¼ medium raw beet

3–4 raw Brussels sprouts

¼ medium raw zucchini

1 raw egg*

2 cups water

stevia to taste

½ tablespoon vanilla bean paste

*Omit the raw egg if you're pregnant or your child is under 12 months. Contrary to popular belief, raw eggs are very healthy, ultra-nutritious, and totally safe to eat as long as they are organic, within the use-by date, and the shell is clean and intact. I have been eating raw eggs in this way for decades and have never once been sick or slightly unwell. I only avoid raw eggs in pregnancy. To test if the shell is intact, gently place the egg in a glass of water and it should not bubble—if it bubbles the shell is porous and should ideally be used in cooking. If you feel unwell after eating eggs in general, omit the egg from recipes.

Talisha Kendell's Recipes

Talisha Kendell, mother of Ariella, developed Little Mashies reusable food pouches (littlemashies.com) inspired by her own journey of ill health. Diagnosed with a severe digestive disease, she healed herself, going against the advice of doctors who wanted to remove her bowel, by cleaning up her diet and using food pouches to transport healthy foods such as bone broths and smoothies. Her daughter's eating habits also improved considerably using the food pouches at mealtimes, with food enthusiastically eaten rather than thrown on the floor.

Talisha says: This is a high-fat smoothie, but it's all good fat so it is perfect for helping little ones who need extra calories. In addition to these great healthy fats, this smoothie is loaded with vitamins, including B, C, and E, and it contains dietary fiber and antioxidants so it packs a punch for those kiddies needing a nutrient boost. For a lighter smoothie, try substituting almond milk for the coconut milk.

Talisha's recipes yield 2 cups (500ml).

. . . .

Coconut Avo Smoothie

1 medium avocado

1 cup full-fat coconut milk

3 teaspoons fresh lime juice

3 tablespoons Greek yogurt

½ cup blueberries

honey to taste*

*Use if child is over 1 year old; otherwise, use maple or rice malt syrup.

Talisha says: This smoothie is great as a healthy treat at a birthday, Christmas party, or social gathering. It's not for everyday use but gosh it's yummy! It can also be frozen and turned into an ice cream. Please note raw cacao is higher in antioxidants, but much stronger and not recommended for babies and young toddlers. Using 1 to 2 teaspoons will be enough for an older toddler, and 1 to 2 tablespoons provides a lovely chocolate taste for a child or adult. However, as an adult, if having a serious chocolate craving, increase the quantity to 5 tablespoons and your taste buds will be rejoicing! But be wary that using raw cacao will give you quite a buzz—so don't use this much if pregnant or breastfeeding, and stick to regular cocoa.

Red Velvet Smoothie

½ cup beet, boiled or steamed until tender

10 strawberries

10 cherries, pitted

raw cacao or cocoa powder (see comments above)

1 cup almond milk

¼ teaspoon vanilla extract

5 ice cubes

Recommended Resources

Numerous books, journal articles, and websites were referenced in the writing of this book. The following websites and books are a collection of my favorites, and those that are the most useful to peruse for additional reading. The full list of resources are available on my website kristinemiles.com.

Fertility

Excellent resources specific to fertility and preconception care include the work of Francesca Naish and Gabriela Rosa. Francesca Naish has written many books and I can personally vouch for Gabriela's expertise as I was able to conceive my daughter using her advice. The following websites and books are a great place to start when it comes to this important topic.

- fertility.com.au (Francesca Naish's website)
- naturalfertilityandwellness.com (Donielle Bekerly's website)

- naturalfertilitybreakthrough.com (Gabriela Rosa's website)
- natural-fertility-info.com
- withgreatexpectation.com
- Holford, Patrick and Susannah Lawson. *Optimum Nutrition Before, During, and After Pregnancy: The Definitive Guide to a Healthy Pregnancy.* Great Britain: Piatkus Books, 2009.
- Naish, Francesca. *Natural Fertility: The Complete Guide to Avoiding or Achieving Conception,* 4th ed. Australia: Sally Milner Publishing, 2004.
- Rosa, Gabriela. *Eat Your Way to Parenthood: The Diet Secrets of Highly Fertile Couples Revealed.* USA: Goko Associate Publishing, 2008. (Available from naturalfertilitybreakthrough.com.)

Pregnancy

Pregnancy is an exciting time full of wonder and an overwhelming amount of information! The following websites and books come highly recommended to assist the process of understanding what is happening during pregnancy and leading toward birth.

- bellybelly.com.au
- birth.com.au
- modernalternativepregnancy.com
- wellnessmama.com
- whattoexpect.com
- Barham-Floreani, Jennifer. *How to Have Well Adjusted Babies,* 2nd ed. Australia: Well Adjusted, 2009.
- Murkoff, Heidi and Sharon Mazel. *What to Expect When You Are Expecting,* 4th ed. New York: Workman Publishing Group, 2008.

Postnatal/Breastfeeding Resources

There are many fantastic resources to support women after birth, including for breastfeeding women. The book I found most useful when I was learning to breastfeed was *Breastfeeding Made Simple* by Nancy Mohrbacher, and those incredibly supportive of the extended breastfeeding journey include Meg Nagle and Pinky McKay. The following websites and books are an excellent starting point for further information.

- breastfeeding.asn.au (Australian Breastfeeding Association)

- kellymom.com

- llli.org (La Leche League International)

- mobimotherhood.org

- pinkymckay.com (Pinky McKay's website)

- themilkmeg.com (Meg Nagle's website)

- Who.int/en (World Health Organization)

- Barker, Robin. *Baby Love: Everything You Need to Know about Your Baby's First Year*. Australia: Pan Macmillan, 2013.

- Mohrbacher, Nancy and Kathleen Kendall-Tackett. *Breastfeeding Made Simple: Seven Natural Laws for Nursing Mothers*, 2nd ed. Oakland, CA: New Harbinger Publications, 2010.

- West, Diana and Lisa Marasco. *The Breastfeeding Mother's Guide to Making More Milk*. USA: McGraw Hill Books, 2009.

Baby and Toddler Resources

The two most useful books regarding feeding children I found were *My Child Won't Eat!* by Carlos Gonzalez, and *Baby-Led Weaning* by Gill Rapley. Though I followed neither book exclusively, I believe understanding the key messages in both books significantly reduces the stress of mealtimes with children. The following websites and books are excellent resources regarding children's feeding, general health, and parenting.

- aaaai.org (American Academy of Allergy, Asthma, and Immunology)

- aap.org (American Academy of Pediatrics)

- allergy.org.au (ASCIA—Australasian Society of Clinical Immunology and Allergy)

- askdrsears.com

- drgreene.com

- kellymom.com

- nhmrc.gov.au (Australian Government—National Health and Medical Research Council)

- pinkymckay.com (Pinky McKay's website)

- scienceofmom.com (Alice Callahan's website)

- Who.int/en (World Health Organization)

- Gonzalez, Carlos. *My Child Won't Eat!: How to Enjoy Mealtimes without Worry*. London: Pinter & Martin Limited, 2012.

- Rapley, Gill and Tracey Murkett. *Baby-Led Weaning: Helping Your Baby to Love Good Food*. United Kingdom: Vermilion, 2008.

- Sunderland, Margot. *The Science of Parenting: How Today's Brain Research Can Help You Raise Happy, Emotionally Balanced Children.* New York: DK Publishing, 2006.

- van de Rijt, Hetty and Frans Plooij. *The Wonder Weeks: How to Stimulate the Most Important Developmental Weeks in your Baby's First 20 Months and Turn these 10 Predictable, Great, Fussy Phases into Magical Leaps Forward.* The Netherlands: Kiddy World Publishing, 2013.

General Health and Nutrition Resources

There is a wealth of information available these days about nutrition and what constitutes a healthy diet, and many opinions exist, making research potentially very confusing. The following websites and books are a great starting point for valuable health and nutritional information.

- chriskresser.com (Chris Kresser's website)

- healthaliciousness.com

- nutritiondata.self.com

- westonaprice.org (The Weston A. Price Foundation)

- whfoods.com (World's Healthiest Foods)

- Campbell-McBride, Natasha. *Gut and Psychology Syndrome: Natural Treatment for Autism, Dyspraxia, A.D.D., Dyslexia A.D.H.D., Depression, Schizophrenia,* 2nd ed. United Kingdom: Medinform Publishing, 2010.

- Gillespie, David. *Toxic Oil: Why Vegetable Oil Will Kill You and How to Save Yourself.* Australia: Viking, 2013.

- Miles, Kristine. *The Green Smoothie Bible: Super-Nutritious Drinks to Lose Weight, Boost Energy, and Feel Great.* Berkeley, CA: Ulysses Press, 2012.

- Miles, Kristine. *Green Smoothies for Every Season: A Year of Farmers Market–Fresh Super Drinks.* Berkeley, CA: Ulysses Press, 2013.

- Perlmutter, David. *Grain Brain: The Surprising Truth about Wheat, Carbs, and Sugar—Your Brain's Silent Killers.* New York: Little, Brown, and Company, 2013.

- Price, Weston. *Nutrition and Physical Degeneration: A Comparison of Primitive and Modern Diets and Their Effects.* United Kingdom: Benediction Classics, 2010.

Conversion Charts

TEMPERATURE CONVERSIONS

FAHRENHEIT (°F)	CELSIUS (°C)
325°F	165°C
350°F	175°C
375°F	190°C
400°F	200°C
425°F	220°C
450°F	230°C

VOLUME CONVERSIONS

U.S.	U.S. EQUIVALENT	METRIC
1 tablespoon (3 teaspoons)	½ fluid ounce	15 milliliters
¼ cup	2 fluid ounces	60 milliliters
⅓ cup	3 fluid ounces	90 milliliters
½ cup	4 fluid ounces	120 milliliters
⅔ cup	5 fluid ounces	150 milliliters
¾ cup	6 fluid ounces	180 milliliters
1 cup	8 fluid ounces	240 milliliters
2 cups	16 fluid ounces	480 milliliters

WEIGHT CONVERSIONS

U.S.	METRIC
½ ounce	15 grams
1 ounce	30 grams
2 ounces	60 grams
¼ pound	115 grams
⅓ pound	150 grams
½ pound	225 grams
¾ pound	350 grams
1 pound	450 grams

Index

physical recovery, 177–78;
  stress, 178–79; swelling, 175
Pouches, reusable, for babies,
  273–74
Powders: lactogenic, 198;
  protein, 24, 266, 290;
  superfood, 24–25, 266
Preconception, 48–103; nutrient
  recommendations, 50–66;
  smoothie recipes, 79–103
Preeclampsia, 119–20
Pregnancy, 104–71; do's and
  don'ts, 105–107; essential
  nutrients, 126–46; and fats,
  40–41; smoothie recipes,
  145–71; symptoms, 108–26
Premature births, 237; and iron
  deficiency, 232
Probiotics, 64–66, 143–44; and
  breast milk, 187–88; for
  children, 266; in smoothies,
  24
Progesterone, 71–74; and
  constipation, 113–14; and
  heartburn, 109; and men, 72
Prolactin, 183, 193
Protein powders, in smoothies,
  24; for children, 266, 290
Proteins, 63–64, 141, 142–43, 178,
  235–36
Pumpkin, in smoothies, 16

Quinoa, in smoothies, 18
Quirky Cooking, 307

Rapley, Gill, 267
Real Treats, 305
Recovery, physical, post-birth,
  177–78
Relaxin (hormones), 114–15
Rice cereal, 250–51
Rice (malt) syrup, in smoothies,
  31

Salmonella risk, 23, 298–99
Saponins, 195; and quinoa, 18
Saturated fats, 34
Secondary plant metabolites, 3
Seeds, 39; and allergies, 256;
  for children, 256–58; in
  smoothies, 21; soaking, 22–23,
  257
Selenium, 54–55, 138, 187
Self-weaning, of baby, 188–89
Serotonin, 193, 282
Serum iron. *See* Iron
Silica, and skin care, 116
Skin care, 116–17; smoothie
  recipes, 161–64
Smoothie recipes: babies/
  toddlers, 294–98, 299–318;
  breast milk quality, 214–17;
  cramps, 164–67; featured,
  305–18; first six weeks [after
  birth], 206–209; first trimester,
  149–55; healthy milk supply,
  226–29; highly lactogenic,
  220–26; immune boosting,
  217–20; liver cleansing,
  92; luteal phase, 97–103;

Toppings, for smoothies, 27
Toxic Oil, 37
Trans fats, 36–37
Tryptophan, 193, 282
Turmeric, in smoothies, 26–27
"2-week wait" period, 78–79
Tyrosine, 282

Urinary frequency, 123–24

Vaginal births, recovery, 177–78
van de Rijt, Hetty, 243
Vanilla, in smoothies, 25
Vegetables, in smoothies, 16–17;
    for children, 254–56; tips, 17
Vegetarianism: and children,
    235–36; and pregnancy, 141
Vitamin A (retinol), 56–57,
    127–28, 186, 236–37
Vitamin B12 (cobalamin), 52–53
Vitamin C, 57–58, 130, 186
Vitamin D, 62, 130, 186, 234–35
Vitamin E (tocopherol), 58,
    131–32, 186

Vitamin K, 132–33
Vomiting. See Nausea

Water, in smoothies, 12–13; for
    children, 260–61
Weaning. See Solids
Weight gain, 120–22
Westwick, Kira, 309–10
Whitton, Jo, 307–308
Wholesome Kids, 309
The Wonder Weeks, 191, 243

Xenoestrogens, 72–73;
    environmental, 195
Xerophthalmia, and vitamin A,
    128

Yogurt, in smoothies, 14–15

Zest, in smoothies, 25
Zinc, 55–56, 138–39, 187, 194,
    233–34

Recipe Index

Acknowledgments

I have so many people to thank in the making of this book.

First, a huge thank you to my publisher, Ulysses Press. Thanks to Keith Riegert, who has been with me since the beginning with the creation of *The Green Smoothie Bible,* and to Katherine Furman and Alice Riegert for this book. This project has been a labor of love for more than two years. *Homemade Smoothies for Mother and Baby* has grown along the same timeline as my child, with its inception while I was newly pregnant, through to my daughter being a toddler. A difficult pregnancy and postnatal period and the sudden passing of my dear mother, have resulted in the most challenging few years of my life. I am eternally grateful for the patience and sympathy extended to me by Keith, Katherine, and Alice during this time. Thank you for trusting in me to complete this work.

Thank you to my wonderful recipe contributors: Alexx Stuart, Franki Hopkins, Jo Whitton, Susan Stock, Kira Westwick, Alison Beresford, Bianca Slade, Sarah Pearce, Amy Semmens, Gabriela Rosa, Kelly Solohub, Sarah Keys, and Talisha Kendell.

Thank you to my superstar recipe testers: Hilary Mann, Susan Stock, Melissa Jenkins, Adrienne Rush, Lien Sim, Lauren Papas, Kara Cassells, Mandy Mercuri, Jennie Smythe, Chloe Arthur, Louise Aracas, Claire Williams, Linzi Harrocks, Claire Hart, Siobhan Leahy,

Natalia Sojak, Kelly Solohub, Kellie Berwick, Elise Parker, and my husband, Ben Miles.

Also thank you to my testimonial providers Megan Eddy, Gabriela Rosa, Hilary Mann, Vicky Douglas, Susan Stock, and those of you with alternative names for reasons of privacy.

And finally to the 300-plus mamas who completed my survey—thank you!

About the Author

Kristine Miles is the author of the best-selling book *The Green Smoothie Bible*, and a physiotherapist of 19 years standing with a special interest in nutrition. She is passionate about life-long learning, eating, cooking, and living a low-toxic lifestyle. Kristine works in private practice and lives by the stunning surf coast of Phillip Island, Australia with her husband and daughter. Her website, www.kristinemiles.com, is a hub for healthy food and smoothie recipes (including Thermomix recipe conversions), smoothie making tips, and natural parenting practice and philosophy. You can sign up for her newsletter and access special offers including product discount codes, and you can also follow Kristine on Facebook (KristineMilesAuthor) and Instagram (kristine_miles).

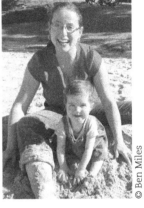

© Ben Miles

CPSIA information can be obtained
at www.ICGtesting.com
Printed in the USA
LVHW020944110222
710695LV00011B/1268